THE FITNESS INSTRUCTOR'S
HANDBOOK

THE FITNESS INSTRUCTOR'S
HANDBOOK

A Professional's Complete Guide to Health and Fitness

MORC COULSON

FIREFLY BOOKS

A FIREFLY BOOK

Published by Firefly Books Ltd. 2007

First printing

Publisher Cataloging-in-Publication Data (U.S.)

Coulson, Morc, 1961–
  Fitness instructor's handbook : a professional's complete guide to health and fitness / Morc Coulson.
[   ] p. : ill. ;   cm.
Includes index.
Summary: Offers a blend of theory and practice on every aspect of health and fitness.
ISBN-13: 978-1-55407-330-6 (pbk.)
ISBN-10: 1-55407-330-8 (pbk.)
  1. Physical fitness–Handbooks, manuals, etc.   2. Exercise–Physiological aspects–Handbooks, manuals, etc.
3. Health. I. Title.
613.7 dc22   GV481.C675   2007

Library and Archives Canada Cataloguing in Publication

Coulson, Morc, 1961-
  Fitness instructor's handbook : a professional's complete guide to health and fitness / Morc Coulson.
Includes index.
ISBN-13: 978-1-55407-330-6
ISBN-10: 1-55407-330-8

  1. Physical fitness–Handbooks, manuals, etc.   2. Exercise–Physiological aspects–Handbooks, manuals, etc.
3. Health. I. Title.

GV481.C675 2007   613.7   C2007-902075-5

Published in the United States by
Firefly Books (U.S.) Inc.
P.O. Box 1338, Ellicott Station
Buffalo, New York 14205

Published in Canada by
Firefly Books Ltd.
66 Leek Crescent
Richmond Hill, Ontario L4B 1H1

Text and cover design: James Watson
Front cover image: © Creasource/Corbis

Printed in the United Kingdom

CONTENTS

FOREWORD

Knowledge and support have helped many a top athlete over the years, not just physiologically but from a psychological, rehabilitative and medical perspective. It is common for individual athletes to use specifically designed programs to train at the correct intensity, in the correct frame of mind and with nutritional advice that enables optimum recovery. There are also many recreational health and fitness participants who could benefit in many ways from support given by suitably qualified people. *The Fitness Instructor's Handbook* offers a comprehensive guide to the theory and practical application of health and fitness knowledge, linked closely to the typical occupational standards in this area. It is hoped that this book will help to develop a culture of education in health and fitness, not just for the benefit of the coach or instructor, but for the entire population.

Steve Cram, MBE and BBC TV
Sports Personality of the Year, 1983

PREFACE

This book has been written as a reference guide for a wide audience, such as those who have an interest in health and fitness and sports, and for individuals who, both now and in the future, are involved in prescribing gym-based cardiovascular and resistance exercise to clients who are apparently healthy, or referred to as "apparently healthy." The main objective of this book is to address the underpinning knowledge related to qualifications in the health and fitness industry and to show how that knowledge can be applied in a practical environment. It was a conscious decision to closely relate the book to health and fitness qualification requirements and learning objectives in order to provide a comprehensive reference guide that would promote the professionalism of the industry.

The chapter topics have been selected to provide complete coverage of the standard required knowledge content for "Instructing Exercise and Fitness Knowledge" and "Instructing Physical Activity and Exercise Knowledge" qualifications. At the start of each chapter are standard criteria related to these fundamental qualifications and the objectives to be addressed. At the end of the chapter you will find review questions relating only to that particular chapter. Answers to these can be found at the back of the book. Each chapter also contains space for review notes and a list of further reading for those who would like to pursue the topic in more depth.

ACKNOWLEDGMENTS

I would like to sincerely thank all who contributed in any way to the development and writing of this book. A big thank you goes out to SkillsActive and REPs for their continuing endeavours in trying to professionalise and bridge the gap between the Health and Fitness industry and academia, and to the many training organisations that are actively embracing this philosophy.

Many thanks to Robert Foss, commissioning editor at A&C Black Publishers, who gave insightful direction throughout, and Lucy Beevor, editor also at A&C Black Publishers, who made the whole process so easy and yet so professional. Thanks also to my colleague Dave Archer, physiologist at the University of Sunderland, who provided a very welcome and needed critical eye, and to the Health and Racquets Club in Sunderland for the use of their facilities. I would like to give a special thank you to all my family for their belief in me and to my lovely wife Lorretta for just being there. Finally, a heartfelt thank you to my brother and friend Graham – if it were not for your support over the years, this would never have happened.

INTRODUCTION

More and more, both governments and society are committed to improving the nation's fitness and health. Organizations such as the President's Council on Physical Fitness and Sports and the Public Health Agency of Canada promote physical activity, fitness and sports, but proper fitness requires the assistance of a properly qualified fitness instructor.

While there is no one body in the United States or Canada that oversees and governs a single, mandatory certification system for fitness instructors, organizations such as the Aerobics and Fitness Association of America, the American Council on Exercise, the YMCA and the Canadian Society for Exercise Physiology offer and oversee their own accredited certification programs.

The fitness industry is continuously evolving and maturing and works closely with various levels of government to help deliver its public health targets and represent the interests of the numerous health and fitness organizations across North America. These include operators from the public and private sectors, service and product suppliers to the industry, training providers, independent professionals and affiliated bodies.

The primary goal is to get more people more active, more often. This can largely be achieved by developing and running high-profile programs designed to encourage people who are not regularly active to visit gyms and fitness centers.

When people who were not previously physically active begin a new fitness program it is crucial they receive proper instruction. Ensuring health and fitness professionals are appropriately skilled and qualified is essential. This includes working with higher and further education institutions to develop qualification frameworks that will enable graduates to leave college or university with industry-recognized vocational qualifications. Safeguarding and promoting the health and interests of people who use the services of exercise and fitness instructors, teachers and trainers is also extremely important. A process of self-regulation that recognizes standard qualifications and practical competency has been developed, and these basic qualifications are broadly outlined below.

Instructors should continue their personal development throughout their career by attending a minimum number of hours each year in the form of further qualifications, workshops, seminars or conferences. This is commonly known as continuing professional development. Below is an overview of "Instructing Exercise and Fitness Knowledge" and "Instructing Physical Activity and Exercise Knowledge" qualifications.

Instructing Exercise and Fitness Knowledge

Three broad categories are covered: gym, exercise to music and aqua. Instructors may be proficient in one or more of these categories. The basic structure of this qualification is outlined below.

Common Mandatory Units	
1	Deal with accidents and emergencies.
2	Evaluate coaching sessions and develop personal coaching practice.
3	Support participants in developing and maintaining fitness.

Common Optional Learning Objectives		
Group Exercise with Music Pair	Gym-based Exercise Pair	Water-based Exercise Pair
Plan and prepare a group exercise with music session.	Plan and prepare a gym-based exercise session.	Plan and prepare a water-based exercise session.
Instruct a group exercise with music session.	Instruct a gym-based exercise session.	Instruct a water-based exercise session.

Instructing Physical Activity and Exercise Knowledge

Qualifications under this category generally relate to instructing physical activity and the relevant exercise knowledge. Most are composed of six learning objectives that cover five knowledge areas, as outlined at right and below.

Common Knowledge Areas	
1	Behavior Change
2	Anatomy
3	Functional Kinesiology
4	Energy Systems
5	Concepts and Components of Fitness

Common Mandatory Learning Objectives	
1	Collect and analyze information to plan a progressive physical activity program.
2	Plan, review and adapt a progressive physical activity program.
3	Plan and instruct specific physical activities.
4	Provide motivation and support to clients during a progressive physical activity program.
5	Apply the principles of nutrition and weight management to a progressive physical activity program.
6	Manage, evaluate and improve own performance in providing physical activity.

Additional qualifications can be gained in the following categories:

	Common Additional Learning Objectives
1	Collect and analyze information to plan a progressive physical activity program.
2	Adapt a physical activity program to the needs of older adults.
3	Adapt a physical activity program to the needs of disabled clients.
4	Adapt a physical activity program to the needs of pre- and postnatal clients.
5	Integrate core stability and flexibility exercises into a physical activity program.
6	Design a physical activity program for children and young people.
7	Adapt a physical activity program to a specific sport.
8	Plan and deliver personal training.
9	Design, agree and adapt a physical activity program with referred patients / clients.
10	Plan, market and sell services.

Qualification types

A very diverse range of organizations, such as private training providers, colleges and universities, deliver fitness instructor qualifications. Delivery may vary with respect to contact time and mode of delivery depending on the provider. As previously mentioned, there is no one central authority overseeing fitness instructor qualifications in the United States or Canada, so it is imperative that would-be student instructors research their options. A number of accredited colleges offer fitness instructor training, and it's also worth exploring the courses offered by reputable organizations, such as your local YMCA. In addition to entry qualifications, there are many courses, seminars, workshops and events available across North America.

PART ONE

THEORETICAL KNOWLEDGE FOR HEALTH AND FITNESS

Part 1 of this book addresses theoretical knowledge for health and fitness. Each chapter provides example questions as well as a list of recommended reading for each chapter should the reader wish to gain a more in-depth knowledge of the relevant topic area.

THE SKELETAL SYSTEM

1

OBJECTIVES

After completing this chapter, you will be able to

1 Describe the structure of bone, in particular long bones.

2 Classify bones and give examples of each type.

3 Describe the process of bone growth, in particular within long bones.

4 Discuss the factors that can affect bone density.

5 Explain the effects of exercise on bone.

6 Describe the structure and list the functions of the skeleton.

7 Identify the major bones in the body.

8 Describe the structure and list the functions of the vertebral column.

9 Describe the structure and function of vertebral and intervertebral disks.

10 Describe the range of motion available at the spine.

11 Describe common postural definitions and list a range of common injuries associated with the spine.

Instructing Exercise and Fitness Knowledge

Basic Anatomy and Physiology

- The structure and function of the skeleton; structure and range of movement of the spine; bone growth.
- The long- and short-term effects of exercise on bone.

Instructing Physical Activity and Exercise Knowledge

Anatomy: Bones

- Five types of bone:
  - Structure and proportion of compact/cancellous bone
  - Typical location/role within the body

- Structure of a long bone:
  - Diaphysis, epiphysis, epiphyseal plate, periosteum, medullary cavity, cartilage, compact bone, cancellous bone
  - Susceptibility to breakage/damage – epiphysis vs diaphysis
- Growth of a long bone:
  - The ossification process: prenatal through childhood to adulthood
  - The role of osteoblasts and osteoclasts
  - Hormonal regulation of bone growth
  - Key nutrients in bone growth
  - Calcium regulation
  - Bone remodeling
  - Osteoporosis
- Names of all major bones:
  - Articulations and joint movements
  - Muscle attachment sites
- The skeletal system (axial and appendicular skeleton):
  - Structure and function of each part
- Structure of the spine; postural deviation:
  - Five curves of the skeleton
  - Number and structure of vertebrae in each section
  - The vertebral foramen
  - Structure and function of vertebral disks
  - Facet joints
  - Kyphosis, lordosis and scoliosis
  - Neutral spine
- The range of medical conditions common in back pain patients that may be aggravated by physical activity or lead to injury.

Introduction

This chapter deals with the anatomic systems of the body, in particular the formation of bone and the skeletal system from the perspective of structure and function, as well as the effects of exercise on these systems. Instructors should be able to identify the components of the skeletal system and describe their functions, as well as describe how exercise can impact on bone growth.

Later chapters provide physiologic and biomechanical principles that, together with the anatomic knowledge covered in this chapter, will provide fitness instructors with the understanding and ability to design appropriate exercise programs for apparently healthy individuals and to understand the effects of various types of exercise on the human body.

Common anatomic terms

As the first part of this book is concerned with the anatomy of the human body, it is useful to understand the terms used to describe it. When using anatomic terms, the body is assumed to be in a position where the arms are resting by the sides of the body with the palms facing forward, with a theoretical line drawn down the center of the body. When the limbs move, the movement is described in reference to this line. Table 1.1 contains some common anatomic terms and their description.

Table 1.1	Common anatomic terms
Term	Description
Anterior	Front
Posterior	Back
Medial	Toward the midline
Lateral	Away from the midline
Superior	Upper
Inferior	Lower
Proximal	Near to
Distal	Away from
Prone	Facing down
Supine	Facing up

Bone

Bone structure

Bone is classified as a calcified connective tissue and, when it is fully developed, is the hardest tissue in the body. In a typical bone there are two types of bone tissue: *compact* and *cancellous*.

Compact bone

Compact bone is also known as *cortical* bone. It has a hard outer layer that provides a strong structure called the *cortex*, which provides protection and support to help resist stresses imposed during movement and weight-bearing activities. It is often assumed that compact bone is solid, but this is not the case: it contains a series of canals through which blood and lymph vessels and nerves pass. This series of canals gives compact bone greater strength than if the bone was completely solid as the canal systems are aligned in the same direction along the lines of stress of each bone, helping to resist fracture.

Cancellous bone

Cancellous bone is otherwise known as *trabecular* bone. Within cancellous bone there is a 'spongy' structure that contains red bone marrow, which is where blood cells are made. This type of bone also contains a series of canals that are larger than those in compact bone as the red bone marrow needs to get a rich blood supply to produce red blood cells.

A double layer of tough, dense collagen fibers about the thickness of a nail, called the *periosteum*, covers most of the surface of bones. It provides attachment for tendons and ligaments and gives protection to the bone.

Classification of bones

Bones are often classified according to their formation and shape. The shape of a bone can sometimes help to identify the role it has in the body. Bone is normally classified into the five groups below (see also Figure 1.1).

1. Long bones

Long bones are found mainly in the limbs and comprise a shaft with two extremities. The shaft is known as the *diaphysis* and the extremities are known as the *epiphyses*. Just before each epiphysis is a region known as the growth plate, or *epiphyseal cartilage*. This is the region in the bone at which growth occurs; when growth finally stops in adulthood the epiphyseal cartilage becomes fully developed bone. Fatty yellow bone marrow is found within the central part of the long bone known as the *medullary canal*. Long bones are attached to muscles that can pull and create movement, so they act as levers to provide locomotion for the body. The femur and humerus are examples of long bones.

2. Short bones

Short bones are designed mainly for lightness and strength. They are usually cube-shaped and are mainly spongy (cancellous) bone with a thin outer layer of compact bone. Examples of short bones are the carpals (wrist) and tarsals (ankles).

3. Flat bones

Flat bones are spongy (cancellous) bones sandwiched between two layers of compact bone. They either give protection, such as in the skull, or provide a large area for muscle attachment, such as in the pelvis.

| Figure 1.1 | **Examples of the different types of bone in the body** |

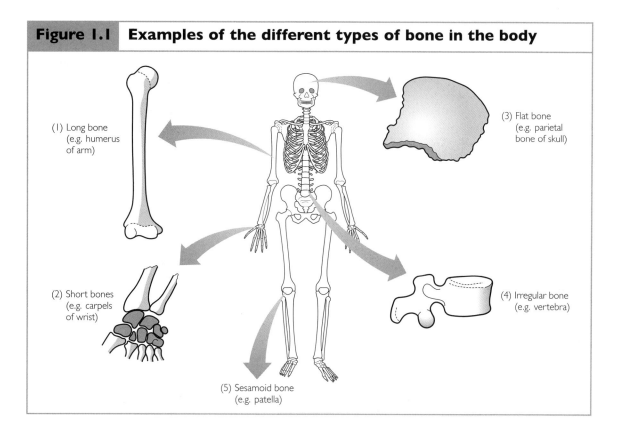

(1) Long bone (e.g. humerus of arm)

(2) Short bones (e.g. carpels of wrist)

(3) Flat bone (e.g. parietal bone of skull)

(4) Irregular bone (e.g. vertebra)

(5) Sesamoid bone (e.g. patella)

4. Irregular bones

Irregular bones usually have bony projections for the purpose of muscle attachment. The vertebrae (bones of the spine) are examples of irregular bones.

5. Sesamoid bones

Sesamoid bones are seed-like bones, normally the size of a pea, that are developed within the tendon of a muscle, such as the patella in the knee joint. Sesamoid bones usually protect tendons from excessive wear and tear. They can also change the direction of pull of a tendon to increase the mechanical advantage at a joint in which the tendon crosses.

TASK

Figure 1.1 shows examples of the five types of bone and where they can be found in the body. Try to identify all of the bones in the skeleton and assign them to one of the five classifications.

Bone growth

Bone growth in humans begins at birth and is not complete until about the 25th year but can, in some cases, be complete around the age of 18. Bones start out in the body as tissues known as cartilage, membrane and tendon until a process called *ossification* (*oss* meaning bone and *fication* meaning to make) gradually replaces these tissues with bone. Certain hormones released within the body, such as *growth hormone*, testosterone, estrogen and calcitonin, help to regulate and control bone development.

Long bones, such as those in the limbs, grow in length at the epiphyseal or growth plate, which is the region near the end of the diaphysis or shaft of the bone (see Figure 1.2). The ends, or epiphyses, of long bones are enlarged and are covered in a tissue called hyaline cartilage (see page 72), which provides protection for the end of the bone.

TASK

Draw and label the parts of a typical long bone and list the functions of each part.

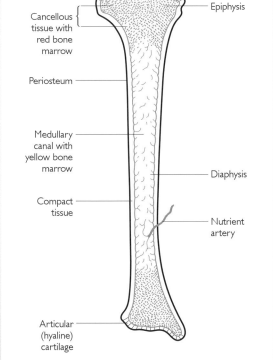

Figure 1.2 The structure of a typical long bone

- Epiphysis
- Cancellous tissue with red bone marrow
- Periosteum
- Medullary canal with yellow bone marrow
- Compact tissue
- Diaphysis
- Nutrient artery
- Articular (hyaline) cartilage

Bone tissue contains several types of cell. An *osteocyte* is the main cell of a fully developed bone. Two other types of bone cell, *osteoblasts* and *osteoclasts*, are responsible for building and modeling the bone in which they are located. Osteoblasts are bone-building cells that are involved in the formation of bone; osteoclasts are very large bone-modeling cells that can break down bone formation by digesting protein and minerals, making the bone less dense and therefore weaker. Throughout life, if homeostasis is achieved, then osteoblasts and osteoclasts work together to keep bone at the optimum thickness. If homeostasis is disrupted, it is possible that one type of bone cell can dominate, resulting in either a thickening or weakening of the bone.

Ossification can start as early as in the womb, where osteoblasts secrete protein (primarily collagen) to initiate the process of calcification by forming a meshwork called the *bone matrix*. Osteoblasts get trapped in the matrix and become osteocytes (main bone cells) as the matrix calcifies and hardens. Other osteoblasts then work outward to increase the length of the bone. At the same time, osteoclasts work to remove excess bone and prevent it from becoming too thick. Osteoblasts and osteoclasts work together at the epiphyses of the bone to form an epiphyseal plate, which is responsible for bone growth. This activity is controlled by many hormones at different stages throughout life; one of the most important is growth hormone, which is secreted by the *pituitary gland*.

During growth, the epiphyseal plate is just a layer of hyaline cartilage. When bones stop growing in length – usually between the ages of 18 and 25 – the hyaline cartilage at the epiphyseal plate is replaced by bone. Even though bones do not grow in length after this stage, they can continue to grow in diameter throughout life.

Factors affecting bone growth

Age, lack of weight-bearing activity, smoking and alcoholism can all lead to a loss of calcium and bone marrow. The cancellous part of the bone, therefore, becomes less dense, making the bone weaker and slower to heal. A severe case of this condition is known as *osteoporosis*, which is more common in females (especially postmenopausal) than males: figures suggest that up to 50 percent of postmenopausal women suffer from the condition. Even though it is thought that osteoporosis is not reversible, many studies have shown that exercise can slow down the rate at which osteoporosis occurs – the pull of muscles on bone and the effects of gravity can lead to an increase in bone density (Baechle, 2000; Wilmore and Costhill, 2004). It is therefore important that some type of resistance training be recommended to people with this condition, although care should be taken due to the risk of bone fracture or breaks.

NEED TO KNOW

 The density of bone can be estimated using a technique known as dual-energy x-ray absorptiometry (DEXA). This technique, which involves a very low dose of photon radiation, can also be used to estimate body-fat percentage.

NEED TO KNOW

 Other hormones that influence bone growth include thyroxine, testosterone, estrogen, calcitonin and parathormone.

Diet also has an impact on bone growth and strength. Almost half the content of bone is made up of the minerals calcium and phosphorus. Calcium is always present in the blood as it has many functions in the body – for example it is required for muscle contraction and bone formation – and normal blood calcium levels are 9–11 mg per 100 ml of blood. If blood calcium levels fall, osteoclasts will break down bone to release calcium into the bloodstream. Therefore, a diet low in calcium can make the bones weaker. About 80 percent of the phosphorus in the body is found in and is responsible for the formation of bones and teeth. It also plays an important part in muscle contraction. Dietary sources include dairy products, meat, fish and beans. Finally, vitamins C and D are also important in the process of bone growth: vitamin C is used in the laying down of collagen to form connective tissue, such as in bone formation, whereas vitamin D is essential for the absorption of calcium and phosphorus from the intestine.

The effects of exercise on bone

Physical activity has been shown to stimulate osteoblasts to secrete protein and initiate the bone-building process as a result of placing force on the bone. This is referred to as the *minimal essential strain*. The exact amount of activity required to start this process is unknown but is thought to be equivalent to one-tenth of the force required to fracture the bone. Forces placed on the bone below this threshold are believed to have no effect. Many studies have also shown a correlation between bone density and the strength of the attached musculature, so it appears that resistance training has a positive effect on bone density. However, the formation of new bone is

relatively slow compared to the rapid loss of bone mineral content as a result of immobility or reduced loading, especially following a period of bed rest.

NEED TO KNOW

In general terms, an increase or decrease in muscle strength will result in a corresponding increase or decrease in bone density.

Short-term effects

There are no actual short-term effects of exercise on the bones; instead, exercise initiates the long-term process described below.

Long-term effects

Placing stress on the bones by engaging in weight-bearing exercise is thought to result in the bone tissue becoming stronger over a period of time. However, care must be taken not to place too much stress or high impact on the bones of children who have not fully matured as this can result in damage to the epiphyseal plate.

Exactly how placing stress on the bones results in stronger bone tissue is still a case for debate. However, it is commonly agreed that resistance or impact exercise places stress on the bones that stimulate this mechanism. It is recommended that adolescents and young adults should engage in some sort of weight-bearing activity to help this process occur, but, as stated above, the amount of stress must be limited.

It is also recommended that older adults engage in some sort of bone-stressing exercise because as we get older the amount of calcium taken out of the bones is greater than the amount of calcium taken in by the bones. This is due to the fact that activity levels and dietary intake of calcium and phosphorus usually reduce, while in postmenopausal women a reduction in hormone levels disrupts the activity of osteoblasts (see page 7). In the long-term, this makes the bones less dense and therefore weaker.

NEED TO KNOW

Astronauts in space can lose as much as 1 percent of bone mass per week due to the lack of gravity.

The skeleton

Structure and functions of the skeleton

The human skeleton contains approximately 206 bones and consists of two parts: the *axial skeleton*, which comprises the skull, the vertebral column (backbone), the ribs and the sternum, and the *appendicular skeleton (appendic* meaning to hang on to), which comprises the shoulder and pelvic girdles and the upper and lower limbs (see Figure 1.3). The skeleton as a whole has many important functions, including

- Providing a framework and shape for the body: the size and shape of the skeleton can determine a person's shape.
- Protecting the vital organs: for example the ribcage protects the heart and lungs.
- Acting as levers for movement on which muscles act. When muscles contract they draw together, and as the ends of muscles are normally attached to bones, one attachment will move toward the other.

- Providing surfaces for the attachment of muscles (via tendons) and ligaments.
- Producing red and white blood cells and platelets. This is the function of the cancellous or 'spongy' bone.
- Storing minerals such as calcium, phosphorus, potassium and sodium.

It is important that health and fitness instructors are familiar with the names and locations of the bones in the body as, together with the muscles, they provide movement and locomotion.

The bones of the shoulder (pectoral) girdle

See Table 1.2 and Figure 1.4. The shoulder or pectoral girdle attaches the arms to the body, or, in other words, the upper limbs to the axial skeleton. It consists of a *scapula* (shoulder blade) and *clavicle* (collar bone) on each side of the body. The scapula has a socket called the *glenoid fossa* or *cavity*, which articulates (joins) with the upper arm (*humerus*) to form the shoulder joint. This is a shallow joint that allows for a large degree of mobility at the expense of stability. The most lateral point of the scapula is called the *acromion process*, which articulates with the clavicle to form the acromioclavicular joint. The distance between the two acromion processes is called the *biacromial distance*.

The bones of the upper and lower arm

See Table 1.3 and Figure 1.5. The humerus is the bone of the upper arm that, along with the glenoid fossa of the scapula, makes the shoulder joint. The distal (far) end of the humerus articulates with the two bones of the lower arm or forearm (with the *radius* at the *capitulum* and with the *ulna* at the *trochlear*) to form the elbow joint.

The bones of the hand and wrist

See Table 1.4 and Figure 1.6. The eight short bones located in the wrist are known collectively as the *carpals*. The bones are held

| Figure 1.3 | The bones of (a) the axial and (b) the appendicular skeleton |

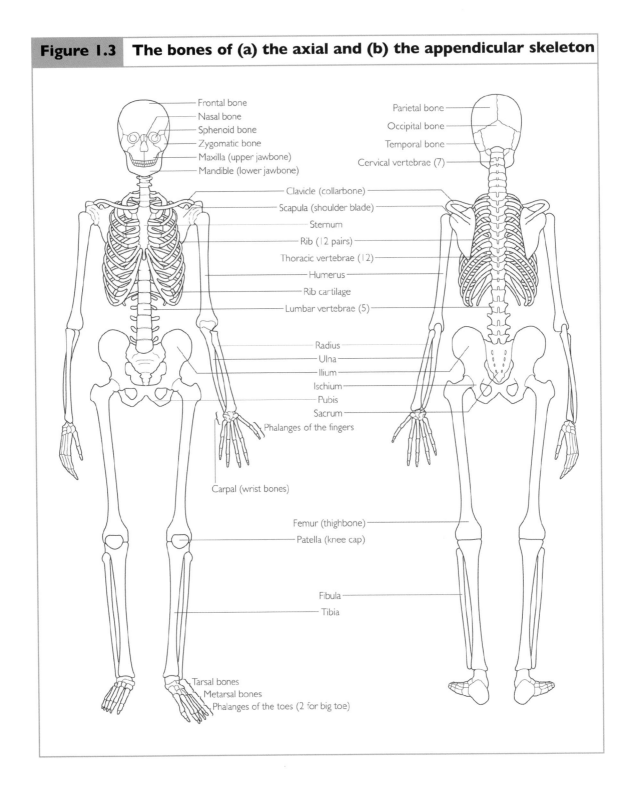

Frontal bone
Nasal bone
Sphenoid bone
Zygomatic bone
Maxilla (upper jawbone)
Mandible (lower jawbone)

Parietal bone
Occipital bone
Temporal bone
Cervical vertebrae (7)

Clavicle (collarbone)
Scapula (shoulder blade)
Sternum
Rib (12 pairs)
Thoracic vertebrae (12)
Humerus
Rib cartilage
Lumbar vertebrae (5)

Radius
Ulna
Ilium
Ischium
Pubis
Sacrum
Phalanges of the fingers

Carpal (wrist bones)

Femur (thighbone)
Patella (knee cap)

Fibula
Tibia

Tarsal bones
Metarsal bones
Phalanges of the toes (2 for big toe)

Table 1.2	The bones of the shoulder girdle	
Bone	Landmark	Description
Scapula	Acromion process	• Projection over the shoulder joint • Site of muscular attachment • Articulates with the clavicle
	Coracoid process	• Projection on the anterior aspect of scapula • Site of attachment for the short head of the biceps
	Spine of the scapula	• Large ridge extending from the acromion process across the posterior surface of the scapula to the medial border of the scapula
	Glenoid fossa	• Shallow depression where the humerus articulates with the scapula
Clavicle	Acromial end	• Articulates with acromion process of the scapula
	Sternal end	• Articulates with the manubrium of the sternum

together tightly by ligaments (see pages 72–74) and have only a small degree of movement. The carpal bones articulate with the ulna and radius to form the wrist joint. At their furthest point, the carpals articulate with five bones in the palm of the hand called the

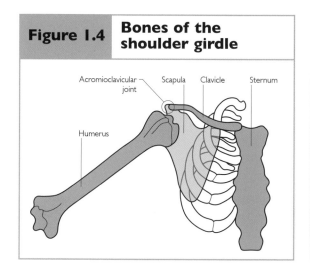

Figure 1.4 Bones of the shoulder girdle

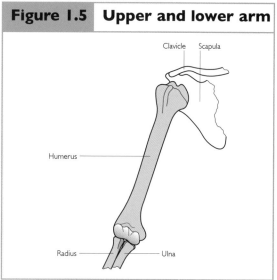

Figure 1.5 Upper and lower arm

Table 1.3	The bones of the upper and lower arm	
Bone	**Landmark**	**Description**
Humerus	Head	• Smooth, round proximal surface that articulates with the glenoid fossa of the scapula
	Humeral condyles (capitulum and trochlear)	• Articular surfaces on the medial and lateral sides of the distal humerus • Capitulum articulates with the head of the radius • Trochlear articulates with the trochlear notch on the ulna
Ulna	Olecranon process	• Process at the proximal end of the ulna • Point of the elbow • Attachment point for the posterior arm muscles
	Head	• Small, partially rounded distal end that articulates with the radius and wrist bones
Radius	Head	• Proximal, drum-shaped end • Articulates with the capitulum of the humerus and the radial notch of the ulna

Table 1.4	The bones of the hand and wrist	
Bone	**Landmark**	**Description**
Carpals	Triquetrum Trapezoid Trapezium Hamate Lunate Capitate Pisiform Scaphoid	• Articulate with the radius and ulna at the proximal side and with the metacarpals at the distal side
Metacarpals		• Short bones located within the palm
Phalanges	Proximal, medial and distal	• Proximal, medial and distal sections allow individual movement for dexterity

metacarpals (*meta* meaning beyond). The metacarpals then articulate with the fingers or *phalanges*, each of which comprises proximal (near), medial (middle) and distal (far) sections, except for the thumb, which has only two sections.

Figure 1.6	**Bones of the hand and the wrist**

Scaphoid

Trapezoid

Trapezium

Capitate

Radius

Ulna

Lunate

Pisiform

Triquetrum

Hamate

Metacarpals

Phalanges

The bones of the pelvic girdle

See Table 1.5 and Figure 1.7. The pelvic girdle provides a strong base to which the axial skeleton attaches via the vertebral column, making a fused joint with the *sacrum*. This is called the *sacroiliac joint*. On each side of the pelvis is a socket called the *acetabulum*, which forms a joint with the femur of the upper leg. This is a deep socket that provides a high degree of stability but has less mobility than the shoulder girdle. The pelvic girdle protects the

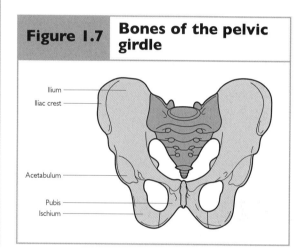

Figure 1.7	**Bones of the pelvic girdle**

Ilium

Iliac crest

Acetabulum

Pubis

Ischium

Table 1.5	The bones of the pelvic girdle	
Bone	Landmark	Description
Ilium		• Large, flat, superior wing-like portion of the pelvis
	Iliac crest	• Large ridge on the superior part of the ilium
Ischium		• Posterior, inferior portion of the pelvis
Pubis		• Anterior, inferior portion of the pelvis
	Acetabulum	• Depression into which the head of the femur articulates

internal organs and in women also provides protection for the fetus during pregnancy. The distance between the two most lateral points is known as the *bicristal distance* and is usually greater in females than in males.

The bones of the upper and lower leg

See Table 1.6 and Figure 1.8. The *femur* (thigh bone) is a long bone in the upper leg and is the longest bone in the body. At the top or head of the femur is a ball-shaped part of the bone that

Table 1.6	The bones of the upper and lower leg	
Bone	Landmark	Description
Femur	Head	• Articulates with the acetabulum of the pelvis
	Greater trochanter	• Large process on the lateral side of the proximal end of bone, to which the gluteal muscles attach
	Condyles	• Rounded medial and lateral smooth articular surfaces where the femur articulates with the tibia
	Intercondylar fossa	• Deep groove between the condyles where the cruciate ligaments attach
	Epicondyles	• Small medial and lateral ridges where the muscles attach
Tibia	Condyles	• Flat, smooth medial and lateral surfaces with which the femur articulates
	Intercondylar eminence	• Crest between the condyles where the cruciate ligaments attach
	Tibial tuberosity	• Knot on the anterior, proximal surface where the patellar ligament attaches
	Medial malleolus	• Large process of the distal, medial aspect of the bone
Fibula	Head	• Proximal enlargement • Articulates with the lateral aspect of the proximal tibia
	Lateral malleolus	• Enlargement on the distal, lateral aspect of the bone
Patella		• Large sesamoid bone in the tendon of the quadriceps muscles of the anterior thigh

articulates with the socket (*acetabulum*) of the pelvis to form the hip joint. At the bottom of the femur are two smooth, rounded surfaces that articulate with the *tibia* to form the *tibiofemoral* or knee joint. Each end of the femur is covered in hyaline cartilage (see page 72).

At the front of the knee joint is a small, triangular sesamoid bone called the *patella* (meaning little dish), which is otherwise known as the knee cap. The patella is located within a band of tendon (see pages 74–75) and glides over the groove on the end of the femur as the knee joint flexes and extends. This is known as the *patellofemoral joint*.

The *tibia* is the main weight-bearing bone in the lower leg and is sometimes known as the 'shin bone.' The top of the tibia is a broad flat surface that articulates with the femur to form the knee joint. The bottom of the tibia articulates with one of the tarsal bones in the ankle, called the *talus*, to form the ankle joint. The *fibula* is a long bone that runs down the lateral side of the tibia and makes a fibrous joint (see page 26) at both ends with the tibia.

The bones of the foot and ankle

See Table 1.7 and Figure 1.9. The seven short bones in the back section of the foot are collectively known as the *tarsals*. The *calcaneus* is the largest of the tarsal bones and is otherwise known as the 'heel bone.' The *talus* is most superior and articulates with the tibia to form the ankle joint. As with the carpals, the tarsal bones are held together tightly by ligaments (see pages 72–74) and have only a small degree of movement.

In the midfoot are five bones known as the *metatarsals* that articulate with the toes, which, like the fingers, are known as *phalanges*. Again, like the fingers, each phalange except for the big

Figure 1.8	**Bones of upper and lower leg**

Head
Neck
Greater tronchanter
Lesser trochanter
Shaft
Femur
Lateral epicondal
Medial epicondal
Knee
Patella (knee cap)
Fibula
Tibia

Figure 1.9	**Bones of the foot and ankle**

Talus
Navicular
Cuneiform (x3)
Metatarsals (x5)
Calcaneus (heel bone)
Cuboid
Phalanges (proximal, medial and distal)

Table 1.7	The bones of the foot and ankle	
Bone	Landmark	Description
Tarsals	Calcaneus talus Cuboid cuneiform (×3) Navicular	
Metatarsals		
Phalanges	Proximal, medial and distal	• Proximal, medial and distal sections allow individual movement and flexibility

toe has three sections: the proximal (nearest), medial (middle) and distal (farthest) phalanges.

The structure and functions of the vertebral column

The spine, otherwise known as the 'vertebral column' or backbone, consists of 24 separate movable bones called *vertebrae* (separated by *intervertebral disks*) and nine fused bones. The movable bones are in three regions – *cervical*, *thoracic* and *lumbar* – and the fused bones are in two regions – *sacrum* and *coccyx* (see Figure 1.10).

The spine is essentially a strong and flexible column that acts as a support system on which the limbs are able to move. Viewed from the side, the structure is curved. The thoracic and sacral regions of the spine are known as primary curves, whereas the cervical and lumbar regions are known as secondary curves. These curves increase the strength of the vertebral column and provide shock absorption during walking, running and jumping.

The top vertebra in the spine is known as the *atlas* and makes a joint with the skull. The bone underneath the atlas is called the *axis* and, along with the atlas, provides a pivot that enables the skull to rotate. The neck region of the spine,

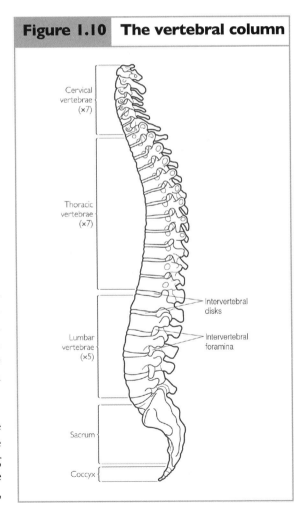

Figure 1.10   The vertebral column

Cervical vertebrae (×7)

Thoracic vertebrae (×7)

Intervertebral disks

Intervertebral foramina

Lumbar vertebrae (×5)

Sacrum

Coccyx

made up of seven bones, is known as the cervical region and allows a degree of movement for the head. Below this, in the upper part of the body, is the thoracic region of the spine, which comprises 12 bones. Here movement is limited as the ribcage is attached to the spine in this region. Below this, in the lower part of the back, is the lumbar spine, made up of five bones. There is a wide range of movement available in this region as this is the part of the spine from which the upper body bends forward and from side to side. The region of the spine known as the sacrum consists of five fused bones and is attached to the pelvis. Finally, the coccyx at the bottom of the spine is made up of four fused bones but really serves no purpose.

As well as attaching the lower part of the body to the upper part, the spine serves many other functions in the body, including

- Protecting the spinal cord – the main nerve stem from the brain, which runs through a hole (*foramen*) in the posterior part of each vertebra.
- Providing access for blood and lymph vessels.
- Allowing certain degrees of movement – each individual vertebra does not have much movement, but the spine as a unit does.
- Providing support for the skull.
- Providing attachment for the ribs and pelvic girdle (the part of the vertebral bodies where the ribs attach to the spine is known as a *facet*).
- Housing shock-absorbing disks.

Vertebral bodies and intervertebral disks

The vertebrae in different regions of the spine can vary slightly in shape and size but essentially share the same features (see Figure 1.11), especially between the second cervical vertebra and the fifth lumbar vertebra. Each vertebra usually has a disk-shaped body with several bony processes that extend from the back of the

Fig. 1.11 A typical vertebral body

Vertebral body
Intervertebral disk
Superior articular process
Spinous process
Transverse process
Spinous process
Lamina
Vertebral foramen
Vertebral body

body, which allow for the attachment of muscles via tendons. At the ends of the bony processes are surfaces known as *facets* that are covered in smooth tissue called *articular cartilage*. The facets of one vertebra make a joint, known as a *zygapophyseal joint*, with the facets of the vertebrae above and below. These joints are synovial (gliding) joints – lubricated with synovial fluid – that allow movement of the spine. The range of motion in each section of the spine mainly depends on the facet joints. The main body of a typical vertebra has an opening on the posterior side known as a *vertebral foramen*, which provides a protective channel through which the spinal cord can run. Nerves branching out from the spinal cord exit from gaps between each adjacent pair of vertebrae.

Between the bodies of adjacent vertebrae are *intervertebral disks* (see Figure 1.12), which provide shock absorption for the spine. The outer layer of the disk, called the *annulus fibrosus* (*annulus* meaning ring-like), is made of cartilaginous fibers and is very tough. The inner part of the disk is called the *nucleus pulposus* (*pulposus* meaning pulp-like) and is made of a soft, viscous, fluid-like material that is very elastic.

Together with the vertebrae, the intervertebral disks provide strong joints in the spine that can withstand a certain amount of compression and

Figure 1.12	A typical intervertebral disk

Intervertebral disk

movement, including *flexion* (bending forward), *extension* (bending backward), *lateral flexion* (bending to the side) and *rotation*. The spine has more movement in the cervical and lumbar regions than anywhere else. Flexion and extension of the spine occur mainly at the lower two lumbar vertebrae; however, there is a limited degree of rotation at the lumbar spine. Flexion and extension are limited in the thoracic spine due to the attachment of the ribs, but there is a reasonable amount of rotation.

Age can decrease the movement available in the spine; it is therefore recommended that mobilization and flexibility exercises make up an important part of an overall exercise program with older adults.

There are many published tables available that provide information about the ranges of motion available at the spine. However, the ranges of motion can differ depending on which author has published the tables; therefore, Table 1.8 shows a typical range of motion for movements of the spine that are common to the published ranges.

stretching. However, it is possible for the outer layer of the disk (the annulus fibrosus) to be ruptured so that the inner part of the disk (the nucleus pulposus) protrudes. This is commonly known as a 'slipped' or herniated disk. It is possible for the nucleus pulposus to exert pressure on a spinal nerve, causing pain either locally or along the length of the nerve.

The disks increase in thickness from the top to the bottom of the spine and can reduce in thickness throughout the day due to the effects of compression and lack of hydration. The disks can return to their original size overnight if hydrated but due to the aging process can degenerate and become thinner as we get older.

Range of movement of the vertebral column

The range of movement between each individual bone in the spine is limited because of the facet joints, as mentioned above. However, the spine as a whole is capable of a wide range of

NEED TO KNOW

The secondary cervical curve develops only after about the first three months of life and the lumbar curve after 12 to 18 months.

Postural definitions

The facet joints and intervertebral disks provide the spine with a certain amount of rigidity, but this is not an adequate amount of support to maintain posture at all times. The muscles provide a certain amount of support, as do the many ligaments that surround the spine. There are two main groups of ligaments related to the spine: the *intrasegmental* and the *intersegmental* ligaments. Like all ligaments, the spinal

Table 1.8	Typical range of motion associated with the spinal column
Movement	Range of motion
Flexion	Total range of 45–55 degrees, mainly at the lumbar region
Extension	Typically 20–35 degrees
Lateral flexion	Up to 60 degrees to either side of the midline, but reducing quickly with age
Rotation	Limited to only a few degrees in the lumbar spine

ligaments allow a certain degree of wanted movement but are designed to prevent unwanted movement.

The small range of motion at the spine where none of the spinal ligaments are placed under any tension is known as the 'neutral zone.' This is considered to be correct alignment or posture for the spine. Postural imbalances can occur where spinal ligaments have been stretched, where spinal muscles are weak or where there are mechanical dysfunctions. Common postural problems include *kyphosis, lordosis* and *scoliosis.*

Kyphosis

This term is used to describe an excessive secondary curve of the thoracic region of the spine. People who suffer from this condition are usually very round-shouldered or hunched in appearance. The diagnosis can often be complicated, but common back-strengthening exercises for the trapezius and rhomboid muscles are normally advocated.

Lordosis

This term describes an excessive primary curve of the lumbar region of the spine. The condition is sometimes referred to as 'sway-back' and is often associated with an increase in abdominal weight, for example in pregnancy or obesity. Core stabilization techniques are usually prescribed as the anterior spinal ligaments can be damaged by this type of posture.

Scoliosis

There are different types of scoliosis, but the term generally refers to a twisting or abnormal curvature of the spine. Scoliosis is normally associated with the thoracic or upper lumbar areas of the spine, although in some cases it can occur in the lower part of the lumbar region. Specific exercises are sometimes effective to rectify muscular imbalance, but they need to be prescribed by a qualified person. For the different types of scoliosis, see Table 1.9.

Common spinal injuries

The spine is a complex mechanical structure and is therefore susceptible to many possible injuries. Injuries can occur in relation to the vertebrae, the spinal ligaments, the intervertebral disks, the spinal muscle and tendons or associated spinal nerves.

Vertebral body injuries

Fractures

Fractures to the vertebral body can be caused as a result of an external blow, known as an *extrinsic* injury, or as a result of internal forces, known as an *intrinsic* injury.

Table 1.9	Types of scoliosis
Scoliosis type	Description
Congenital	This type of congenital deformity is quite rare
Neuromuscular	Due to muscle weakness or imbalance, it is possible for the spine to be pulled to one side
Degenerative	Due to the aging process, it is possible for the spine to develop scoliosis
Idiopathic	This type of scoliosis normally develops in adolescence and usually has no known cause

Spondylolysis

This term refers to the degenerative destruction of the vertebral bodies. The term spondylosis usually refers to a different stage of the same condition.

Spondylolisthesis

This term is used in the case of anterior or posterior sliding of one vertebral body over another. In some cases the stress placed on the vertebral body can cause it to fracture.

Ligament injuries

Ligament tissue has only a slight degree of elasticity as its main function is to provide support. If the movement of the spine takes one of the numerous ligaments of the spine beyond its individual elastic limit, it could result in damage to the ligament. Tears of the ligament are known as *sprains*, whereas the term *rupture* is used to describe a ligament that has completely snapped.

Disk injuries

The term 'disk lesions' refers to an injury of the intervertebral disks. The most common is disk protrusion or herniated disk, where the inner part of the disk (nucleus pulposus) pushes through the outer part of the disk (annulus fibrosis), which can in turn make contact with nerves and cause pain (see also pages 17–18).

Muscle and tendon injuries

Many muscles attach to the spinal column via tendons. Both muscle and tendon tissue can only withstand a certain amount of force, after which injury can occur. As with ligaments, tears in muscle or tendon are known as strains, whereas the term rupture is used for a muscle or tendon that has completely snapped.

Nerve injuries

Nerves that protrude from the spinal column are sometimes disturbed by other structures, such as a protrusion from the intervertebral disk, a narrowing of the spinal foramen or just a muscular spasm. Whatever the cause, any disturbance of a nerve will cause pain. This pain can either be localized or radiate away from the cause of the disturbance. The pain is sometimes given a name that relates to the origin of the nerve that is disturbed; for example 'sciatic pain' radiates down the leg through the sciatic nerves.

TASK

List the common spinal injuries and give a brief description of each.

EXAMPLE QUESTIONS

1.1   The ulna is an example of which type of bone?
   a) Long bone
   b) Short bone
   c) Flat bone
   d) Irregular bone

1.2   The patella is an example of which type of bone?
   a) Long bone
   b) Short bone
   c) Flat bone
   d) Sesamoid bone

1.3   The pelvis is an example of which type of bone?
   a) Long bone
   b) Short bone
   c) Flat bone
   d) Sesamoid bone

1.4   What is the name for the shaft of a long bone?
   a) Epiphysis
   b) Diaphysis
   c) Periosteum
   d) Cancellous

1.5   Which two regions of the spine are primary curves?
   a) Cervical and thoracic
   b) Thoracic and lumbar
   c) Thoracic and sacrum
   d) Lumbar and cervical

EXAMPLE QUESTIONS cont.

1.6 Which two regions of the spine are secondary curves?

a) Cervical and thoracic

b) Thoracic and lumbar

c) Thoracic and sacrum

d) Lumbar and cervical

1.7 Tendons attach to a layer of tissue covering a bone. What is this covering called?

a) Osteoclast

b) Diaphysis

c) Epiphyseal plate

d) Periosteum

1.8 What are the cells in the bone that are responsible for bone-building called?

a) Cancellous cells

b) Osteoblast cells

c) Osteoclast cells

d) Ossification cells

1.9 What are the cells in the bone that are responsible for breaking down bone called?

a) Cancellous cells

b) Osteoblast cells

c) Osteoclast cells

d) Ossification cells

1.10 Which two regions of the spine are capable of the most movement?

a) Cervical and thoracic

b) Thoracic and lumbar

c) Thoracic and sacrum

d) Lumbar and cervical

EXAMPLE QUESTIONS cont.

1.11 What is the outer part of an intervertebral disk called?
 a) Annulus fibrosus
 b) Nucleus pulposus
 c) Epiphyseal plate
 d) Periosteum

1.12 What is the inner part of an intervertebral disk called?
 a) Annulus fibrosus
 b) Nucleus pulposus
 c) Epiphyseal plate
 d) Periosteum

Further reading

Abrahams, P., Craven, J. and Lumley, J. (2005) *Illustrated Clinical Anatomy*, Hodder Arnold

Baechle, R.T. (2000) *Essentials of Strength Training and Conditioning* (2nd ed.), Human Kinetics

Norkin, C.C. and White, D. J. (1995) *Measurement of Joint Motion: A guide to goniometry*, F.A. Davis

Porter, S. (2002) *The Anatomy Workbook*, Butterworth Heinemann

Sewell, D., Watkins, P. and Griffin, M. (2005) *Sport and Exercise Science: An Introduction*, Hodder Arnold

Tortora, G.J. and Grabowski, S.R. (2003) *Principles of Anatomy and Physiology* (10th ed.), Wiley

Wilmore, J.H. and Costhill, D.L. (2004) *Physiology of Sport and Exercise* (3rd ed.), Human Kinetics

Wilson, K.J.W. and Waugh, A. (1998) *Ross and Wilson Anatomy and Physiology in Health and Illness*, Churchill Livingstone

NOTES

JOINTS

2

OBJECTIVES

After completing this chapter, you will be able to

1 List the different classifications of joints and give examples of each.

2 Distinguish between different types of joints by relating to their range of movement.

3 List and give examples of the different types of synovial joints.

4 Identify the common movements within each type of synovial joint.

5 Identify the typical structures within a synovial joint.

Instructing Exercise and Fitness Knowledge

Basic anatomy and physiology

- The structure and function of a synovial joint; range of motion of major synovial joints.

- The long- and short-term effects of exercise on synovial joints.

Instructing Physical Activity and Exercise Knowledge

Anatomy: Joints

- Three types of joints (fibrous, cartilaginous, synovial):
  - The characteristics of each joint
  - Examples of each joint
  - Stability vs movement within each type of joint

- Structure of synovial joints
  - Ligaments, articular cartilage, joint cavity, synovial membrane, synovial fluid
  - Structure and movement potential/anatomic limitations of major joints (shoulder, hip and elbow)
  - Different types of synovial joints and their movement potential

- Names of all major bones
  - Articulations and joint movements
  - Muscle attachment sites

> ■ Joint actions (flexion, extension, hyperextension, adduction, abduction, elevation, depression, lateral flexion, horizontal flexion and extension, plantar flexion, dorsiflexion, internal and external rotation, circumduction, pronation, supination, eversion, inversion)

Introduction

This chapter deals with the anatomic system of the body, in particular the classification of joints within the skeletal system from a perspective of structure, function and the effects of exercise. Instructors should be able to list the classifications of joints and describe the common structures in each type of joint, as well as describe how exercise can affect joints.

Later chapters provide physiologic and biomechanical principles that, together with the anatomic knowledge covered in this chapter, provide the instructor with the understanding and ability to design appropriate exercise programs for apparently healthy individuals and to understand the effects of various types of exercise on the human body.

Basic types of joint

A simple definition of a joint is the articulation or place where two or more bones meet. In other words, a joint is the place where bones come together. Joints are normally classified according to their structure and function, and there are three broad types: *fibrous, cartilaginous* and *synovial.* Fibrous and cartilaginous joints contain connective tissue that binds bone together, whereas synovial joints have a fluid-filled capsule, but no connective tissue, binding the joint. Joints can also be classified according to their degree of movement: they can be *nonmovable,* such as the plates of the skull, which are fused together; *slightly movable,* such as the vertebrae of the spine; or *freely movable,* such as the hip or shoulder.

Joint classification

Fibrous joints

Fibrous joints, sometimes referred to as fixed joints, are made up of immovable interlocking bones that are connected by tissue fibers. These fibers are mainly made up of collagen, a common tissue in the human body. A joint with bones that are able to move in some way is called an *articulated* joint; therefore, a fibrous or fibro joint is a *nonarticulating* joint. An example of this type of joint is the skull.

Fibrous joints need to be very strong to prevent movement of any sort, such as in the joint between the pelvis and the sacrum of the spine (see page 13. This type of joint is also known as a *suture.*

Cartilaginous joints

This type of joint has slightly movable bones surrounded by ligaments that strap the joint together, as they do in other joints. Between the ends of the bones that form the joint are pads of *cartilage,* which can be compressed to allow a small degree of movement. Cartilaginous joints therefore allow a certain amount of movement but also provide a degree of stability. The vertebral bodies and pubis symphysis (pubic bone) are examples of cartilaginous joints.

Synovial joints

Synovial joints are also referred to as freely movable joints as they allow a great deal of movement, with the ligament straps providing most of the support. Unlike the other types, these joints contain a synovial cavity between the articulating bones that allows the range of movement mentioned above. Synovial joints also have a synovial membrane, which can secrete synovial fluid between the bones in the joint to lubricate the articulating surfaces and prevent friction.

TASK

List the three classifications of joint and briefly describe each one in relation to its structure.

Types of synovial joint

There are several types of synovial joint in the body, and they are classified according to their movement or shape. The types of synovial joint in the human body are as follows (see Chapter 3, The Muscular System, for information on the movements):

Ball and socket joints

As the name suggests, this type of joint consists of a ball-like end of one bone coming together with a cup-like end of another bone (see Figure 2.1), for example in the shoulder and hip joint. A large degree of movement in all three planes is available in this type of joint: flexion, extension, abduction, adduction, rotation, pronation, supination, inversion, eversion and circumduction.

Figure 2.1 Ball and socket joint

Head of humerus

Scapula

Hinge

In this type of joint, the convex end of one bone fits into the concave end of another bone (see Figure 2.2). As the name suggests, the joint has

Figure 2.2 Hinge joint

Humerus

Ulna

a motion similar to the hinge on a door – essentially opening and closing – and examples include the elbow, knee and ankle. Only flexion and extension in one plane of movement about a single axis are possible in a joint of this kind.

Gliding or plane joint

The articulating surfaces of these particular joints are usually flat or slightly curved, for example the joints made by the carpal and tarsal bones, and the two surfaces glide over each other (see Figure 2.3). The main movements of gliding joints are side to side and backward and forward.

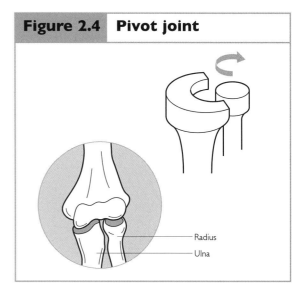

| Figure 2.3 | Gliding or plane joint |

Carpels

Pivot joint

In this particular joint there is usually a rounded or pointed surface of a bone that articulates with a ring-like surface of another bone, for example the radioulnar and cervical spine (see Figure 2.4). The movement is rotational in one axis only.

| Figure 2.4 | Pivot joint |

Radius
Ulna

NEED TO KNOW

The name *synovial* means egg-like as synovial fluid resembles uncooked egg white.

Saddle and condyloid joint

In saddle and condyloid joints such as the thumb, concave and convex surfaces similar to a rider in a saddle fit together to allow movement in two axes, such as side to side and up and down (see Figure 2.5). Movements include flexion, extension, abduction, adduction and circumduction.

Figure 2.5	Saddle and condyloid joint

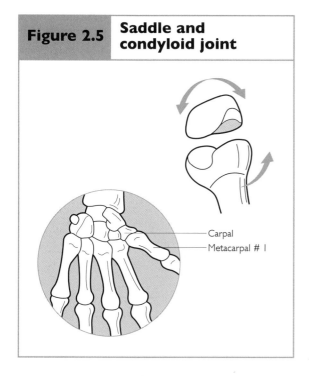

Carpal
Metacarpal # 1

Typical structure of a synovial joint

All synovial joints in the body have particular characteristics in common (see Figure 2.6).

Figure 2.6	A typical synovial joint

Bone
Capsule
Articular cartilage
Synovial fluid
Synovial membrane
Bone

Hyaline or articular cartilage

This covers the ends of the bones that form the joint, providing smooth moving surfaces to prevent friction.

Capsular ligaments

These 'strap-like' collagen fibers hold bones together to provide support but also to allow wanted movement.

Synovial membrane

This secretes synovial fluid, which lubricates the articular cartilage in the joint.

Joint capsule

The joint capsule consists of two layers to provide stability to the joint. The outer layer is a tough fibrous material made up of collagen and elastic fibers and is continuous with the periosteum of the articulating bones. The inner layer is the synovial membrane, which is described above.

Synovial fluid

As well as lubricating the joint surfaces, the synovial fluid contains white blood cells, which remove cellular debris, and nutrients, which nourish the articular cartilage. The synovial fluid becomes less viscous (thick) during activity, so mobilization of the joints prior to intense activity is important.

Proprioceptors

There are many receptors in the cartilage and ligaments that provide information to the central nervous system regarding position and alignment.

The effects of exercise on joints

Short-term effects

During exercise, the synovial membrane secretes synovial fluid into the joint in order to lubricate the bony surfaces and thus prevent friction. This is one of the reasons why it is important to carry out mobilization exercises prior to the main activity so that the joint can be lubricated before any high-impact or high-intensity exercise is undertaken.

Long-term effects

Over time, high-impact and high-intensity exercise can damage the hyaline (articular) cartilage that protects the ends of the bones. If this occurs, there may be some damage to the bone itself, resulting in a condition known as *osteoarthritis*. This can cause inflammation and pain within the joint.

Damage to ligament tissue is common as ligament has only a limited range of elasticity (up to 6 percent). As blood supply to the ligaments is very poor, the tissues can take a very long time to heal; during the healing process the stability that the ligaments normally provide to the joint can be impaired.

TASK

List and describe the typical structures within a synovial joint.

EXAMPLE QUESTIONS

2.1 The tibia and the fibula make what type of joint?

a) fixed

b) cartilaginous

c) synovial

d) hinge

2.2 The pelvis and the sacrum make what type of joint?

a) fixed

b) cartilaginous

c) synovial

d) hinge

2.3 The pelvis and the femur make what type of joint?

a) fixed

b) cartilaginous

c) synovial

d) hinge

2.4 The atlas and the axis make what type of joint?

a) fixed

b) cartilaginous

c) synovial

d) hinge

2.5 Which of the following is classed as a hinge joint?

a) shoulder

b) hip

c) ankle

d) wrist

EXAMPLE QUESTIONS cont.

2.6 Which two movements are available at a hinge joint?
a) pronation and supination
b) flexion and extension
c) adduction and abduction
d) inversion and eversion

2.7 Which of the following make a joint?
a) femur and radius
b) ulna and tibia
c) sacrum and coccyx
d) phalanges and carpals

2.8 Which of the following make a joint?
a) femur and ulna
b) ulna and radius
c) sacrum and cervical
d) phalanges and tarsals

2.9 Which of the following make a joint?
a) humerus and ulna
b) fibula and radius
c) coccyx and cervical
d) ulna and tarsals

2.10 Which of the following make a joint?
a) tibia and fibula
b) pelvis and radius
c) sacrum and thoracic
d) carpals and tarsals

EXAMPLE QUESTIONS cont.

2.11 Which of the following makes a gliding joint?
 a) tibia and fibula
 b) pelvis and femur
 c) scapula and radius
 d) bones of the carpals

2.12 Which of the following makes a pivot joint?
 a) tibia and fibula
 b) ulna and radius
 c) cervical and thoracic
 d) carpals and tarsals

Further reading

Abrahams, P., Craven, J. and Lumley, J. (2005) *Illustrated Clinical Anatomy*, Hodder Arnold

Baechle, R.T. (2000) *Essentials of Strength Training and Conditioning* (2nd ed.), Human Kinetics

Norkin, C.C. and White, D.J. (1995) *Measurement of Joint Motion: A guide to goniometry*, F.A. Davis

Porter, S. (2002) *The Anatomy Workbook*, Butterworth Heinemann

Sewell, D., Watkins, P. and Griffin, M. (2005) *Sport and Exercise Science: An Introduction*, Hodder Arnold

Tortora, G.J. and Grabowski, S.R. (2003) *Principles of Anatomy and Physiology* (10th ed.), Wiley

Wilson, K.J.W. and Waugh, A. (1998) *Ross and Wilson Anatomy and Physiology in Health and Illness*, Churchill Livingstone

NOTES

THE MUSCULAR SYSTEM

3

OBJECTIVES

After completing this chapter, you will be able to

1 Describe the differences between the three types of muscle.

2 Describe the construction of skeletal muscle.

3 Explain the process of muscle contraction and the sliding filament theory.

4 Distinguish between the properties of fast- and slow-twitch muscle fibers.

5 List and explain the types of muscle contraction.

6 Locate the major muscle groups in the body.

7 List and describe the movements available within the body.

8 Explain the different roles of muscle in the body.

9 Explain what is meant by agonist–antagonist muscle pairing.

10 List and explain the planes of movement of the body.

Instructing Exercise and Fitness Knowledge

Basic Anatomy and Physiology

■ The types of muscular contraction; the location and action of the major muscle groups; how voluntary muscles contract.

■ Long- and short-term effects of exercise on muscles.

Instructing Physical Activity and Exercise Knowledge

Anatomy: Muscles

■ Three types of muscle (cardiac, smooth, skeletal)

  • Cardiac

    • The myocardium

    • Myocardial ischemia – immediate impact of lack of oxygen

    • Oxygen delivery to the myocardium during exercise

- • Smooth
  - • Autonomic nervous system regulation
  - • Controlling blood pressure
- • Skeletal
  - • Structure and function of skeletal muscle (to include epimysium, perimysium, endomysium)
  - • Collagen
  - • Proprioceptors and their function (muscle spindle cells, Golgi tendon organs)
  - • Muscle fiber types
- ■ Names of all major muscles and their origin and insertion
- ■ Muscle shape and actions
  - • Fiber direction and role of muscle
- ■ Muscle contraction
  - • The motor unit
  - • Axon terminals, acetylcholine, sodium ions, the action potential, the sodium–potassium pump
  - • The sliding filament theory to include sarcoplasmic reticulum, calcium ions, adenosine triphosphate
  - • All-or-none law of muscle physiology
  - • Muscle fatigue and oxygen debt
- ■ Types of muscle contraction (concentric, eccentric, isometric, isotonic, isokinetic)
- ■ Joint actions and muscle contraction
- ■ Agonists, antagonists, synergists and fixators applied to a range of exercises
- ■ Delayed-onset muscle soreness
- ■ Three anatomic axes and planes
  - • Explain/label each plane and be able to describe movement in relation to the plane

Introduction

This chapter deals with the muscular system of the body, in particular the skeletal muscle system, from a perspective of structure, function and the effects of exercise. Instructors should be able to list the three types of muscle tissue in the human body and describe the way in which skeletal muscle contracts.

Later chapters provide physiologic and biomechanical principles that, together with the anatomic knowledge covered in this chapter, provide the instructor with the understanding and ability to design appropriate exercise programs for apparently healthy individuals and to understand the effects of various types of exercise on the human body.

Types of muscle

There are three types of muscle tissue in the body: cardiac, smooth and skeletal.

Cardiac muscle (myocardium)

The word 'cardiac' refers to the heart; therefore, only the heart contains cardiac muscle. The cardiac muscle contains protein filaments called *actin* and *myosin* (see pages 39–40), as does skeletal muscle tissue, but the fibers in cardiac muscle are shorter than those in skeletal muscle. The actin and myosin protein filaments in the myocardium are arranged in disk-shaped cells that allow electrical signals to pass between the cells in order to make the heart contract.

The cardiac muscle is described as *involuntary* as no conscious thought is needed to make it contract. Contraction is initiated subconsciously by the *sinoatrial node* (SA node), which is located in the right atrium of the heart. The SA node automatically generates its own impulses that cause an electrical stimulus to spread across the heart via a network of specialist fibers. This then stimulates the ventricles to contract and pump blood into the arteries (see Chapter 7). The SA node is often known as the 'pacemaker.'

NEED TO KNOW

Pacemakers are electrical devices that are fitted to the heart to make it beat when the SA node does not function correctly. Pacemakers can automatically speed up the heart during exercise.

Due to the large number of *mitochondria* (organelles in the cardiac muscle, which use oxygen to produce energy; see Chapter 6), the myocardial cells can contract only aerobically. The cells contain large numbers of *myoglobin* (which carries oxygen) and are red in color. The myocardium extracts a large percentage of

oxygen from the blood compared with skeletal muscle. As a result, during exercise the heart has to pump more blood to supply the increased demand.

The blood flow to the heart can be reduced due to a number of reasons, for example blockages in the blood vessels. A reduced flow of blood to the heart – known as *myocardial ischemia* (*ische* meaning to obstruct and *emia* meaning in the blood) – leads to reduced oxygen delivery (*hypoxia*), from which the cardiac muscle cells can die. Individuals who suffer from reduced blood flow to the heart sometimes experience severe pain in the chest, neck or left arm in a condition known as *angina pectoris*, which translates as 'strangled chest.' Hypoxia can eventually lead to a heart attack (known as a *myocardial infarction*) and even death. If an individual suffers from any condition that limits blood supply (*atherosclerosis*), it follows that high-intensity exercise could potentially create a problem for that individual.

NEED TO KNOW

Once cardiac muscle tissue has died it cannot be regenerated by the body. Therefore, the heart becomes weaker.

Smooth muscle

Found in the walls of hollow internal structures such as the digestive system, smooth muscle automatically controls the movement of the internal systems of the body. As with other muscle tissue, smooth muscle contains actin and myosin protein filaments, but these are not as regular as they are in skeletal muscle. Smooth muscle also contracts more slowly than skeletal muscle and maintains its contraction for longer periods. The proteins in smooth muscle are also more elastic than other muscle types.

When smooth muscle contracts, it can cause narrowing of the structures it surrounds. These include the digestive, circulatory, urinary and reproductive systems. Like cardiac muscle, smooth muscle is described as involuntary as its action is controlled by the autonomic nervous system (without conscious thought). For more on the nervous system, see Chapter 5.

NEED TO KNOW

 Unlike skeletal and cardiac muscle, smooth muscle has considerable powers of regeneration.

Skeletal muscles

Skeletal muscles are normally attached from bone to bone via tendons to provide movement of the body. They are described as *voluntary* as the movement is initiated deliberately.

More than 40 percent of the male body weight is made up of skeletal muscle tissue. The largest of this type of muscle in the body is the gluteus maximus, which is the main part of the buttock. The strongest is usually considered to be the quadricep group, even though the jaw can create a greater force. The longest is the sartorious, which runs from the iliac spine in the pelvis to the medial aspect of the tibia (top of the shin bone).

Skeletal muscles

Skeletal muscle will be covered in more detail as this will be the focus of most exercise

programs, although cardiac muscle can also become stronger as a result of cardiovascular exercise.

Types of skeletal muscle

Skeletal muscles have many different shapes, but they can be broadly categorized into the following shape groups: parallel, pennate and convergent (see Figure 3.1).

Parallel muscles

An example of this type of muscle is the biceps brachii in the arm, where the muscle fibers run parallel to the long axis of the muscle. In other words, the fibers run almost in a straight line from the origin to insertion. Muscles of this type are normally associated with a large range of motion.

Pennate muscles

There are two types of pennate muscle: unipennate and bipennate. Both types of muscle have a central tendon for fiber attachment that runs the length of the muscle. In a unipennate muscle the fibers attach to one side of the tendon only, whereas in a bipennate muscle the fibers attach to both sides. The fibers in all pennate muscles attach at an oblique angle and therefore have less range of motion than parallel muscles.

Convergent muscles

As the name suggests, convergent muscles have a broad origin of fiber connection that then converges to a narrow insertion. This can be seen in muscles such as the pectorals and deltoids. The range of motion in these muscles is limited, but force generation can be quite high.

Figure 3.1 — Examples of skeletal muscle shapes

Convergent

Parallel

Pennate

Structure of skeletal muscle

Skeletal muscle is mainly made up of several types of protein. The main proteins that are responsible for contraction are called *actin* and *myosin*. Actin proteins are bound together to make thin filaments, whereas myosin proteins are bound together to make thicker filaments. As can be seen in Figure 3.2, the thick myosin filaments have protruding heads called *cross-bridges*. These cross-bridges 'grab hold' of the actin filaments and pull them in to cause muscle contraction, using the chemical ATP as energy to do so (see also page 44).

In the muscle, each myosin filament is surrounded by actin filaments. These protein filaments group together to form a *myofibril*, which is the smallest muscle fiber (sometimes referred to as a muscle cell). The protein filaments within a muscle fiber do not run the entire length of the muscle, but are arranged in sections called *sarcomeres*. These are the smallest units able to contract in the muscle. When the sarcomeres are laid end to end the muscles have a striped or striated appearance. This can be seen in Figure 3.2: where the actin and myosin filaments are in rows, the muscle appears darker, but where the myosin filament has no actin filaments around it, the muscle appears lighter. Like all muscles, skeletal muscles have a good blood supply and nerve fibers to pass on the signal to contract (see Muscle contraction, pages 42–44).

Each muscle fiber is surrounded by a sheath of fibrous tissue membrane or *fascia* (meaning bandage) called *endomysium* (*endo* meaning within). This is similar to a sausage wrapped in a skin. The main protein in fascia is called *collagen*. Muscle fibers are then grouped together in a bundle (*fascicle*) and surrounded by another sheath called the *perimysium* (*peri* meaning around). Finally, another sheath called the *epimysium* (*epi* meaning upon) surrounds the entire muscle. At each end of the muscle, the three types of sheath taper off and converge to form an attachment to the bone. These attachment points are called *tendons*. See Figure 3.3.

Figure 3.2 | Actin and myosin filaments

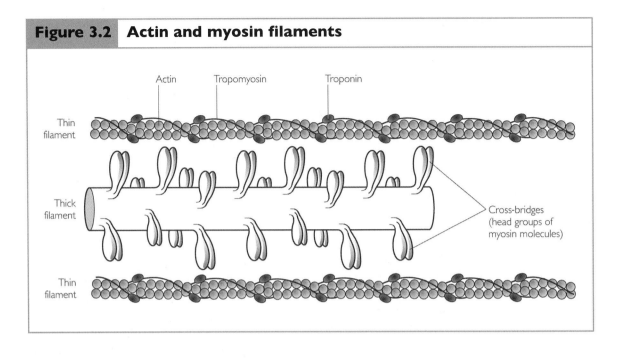

Figure 3.3 | A typical muscle structure

There are also other structures within the muscle, such as *muscle spindles* and *Golgi tendon organs* (GTOs), which have specific roles. These two particular types of structure are known as *proprioceptors*, which refers to the way in which information regarding the position of the various body parts is relayed to the brain.

Muscle spindles

These specialist cells are sensory receptor cells located deep within the muscles. They relay information to the brain concerning the length of a muscle and the speed at which it stretches. If the muscle in which the spindle is located stretches too fast or too far, the muscle spindle causes a reflex action, making the muscle contract to prevent it from becoming damaged. In other words, it causes a built-in safety device known as the *stretch reflex*. The level at which the reflex is initiated is constantly being reset by the brain.

It is also important to note that when the muscle in danger of overstretching contracts as a result of the stretch reflex, the opposing muscle (antagonist) allows it to do so by receiving a signal not to contract. This system is called *reciprocal innervation*.

Golgi tendon organs

These are sensory receptors that lie within the tendon near its junction with a muscle. GTOs are capable of sensing tension in the tendon as a result of muscular contraction or excessive stretching. If this tension exceeds a certain threshold (set by the brain), a reflex operates that causes the muscle responsible for the tension to relax. This is known as the *tendon reflex*.

NEED TO KNOW

An example of the stretch reflex is a doctor tapping her patient's knee with a small hammer. The tendon of the quadriceps is tapped, causing the muscle to stretch quickly. The stretch reflex then causes the quadriceps to contract quickly to prevent any danger.

When skeletal muscles connect to bone, the attachments are known as the *origin* and *insertion*. The origin is the attachment point nearest (proximal) to the midline of the body; the insertion is the attachment point furthest (distal) from the midline. Every muscle has its own nerve supply and is stimulated to contract by the brain sending an electrical impulse or *twitch*. All muscles are in a state of readiness to contract or respond to a signal from the brain. This state of tension has been described as *tone*. By exercising on a regular basis, the amount of muscle tone in the body can be increased, as can the size of a muscle; this is known as *hypertrophy* (*hyper* meaning excessive and *trophy* meaning nourishment). The opposite of this, muscle shrinkage, is known as *atrophy*.

Following a period of strenuous exercise it is common for skeletal muscles to become sore. This soreness, associated with postexercise self-perception, has been termed *delayed-onset muscle soreness* (DOMS). Even though the exact mechanism of this soreness is not fully understood, scientists have found that following periods of intense exercise there is considerable damage at a microscopic level, which may be related to DOMS.

Muscle contraction

The main function of skeletal muscle is to provide movement for the body through contraction. When a muscle contracts, the protein filaments within the muscle fiber slide over one another with the aid of small projections or cross-bridges. This is known as the 'sliding filament' theory (see Figure 3.4).

Several steps occur before the proteins actually move over each other to cause muscle contraction:

1. The brain sends an electrical signal (or 'action potential') to the muscle fiber via a pathway or nerve known as a *motor neuron* (see Figure 3.5). The motor neuron has long branches called *axons* down which the electrical signals can travel. Each motor neuron can make connections with many muscle fibers, depending on the role of the muscle: in the small muscles of the eye, the motor neuron might make connection with only a few muscle fibers, whereas in the

---

Figure 3.4 **The 'sliding filament' theory**

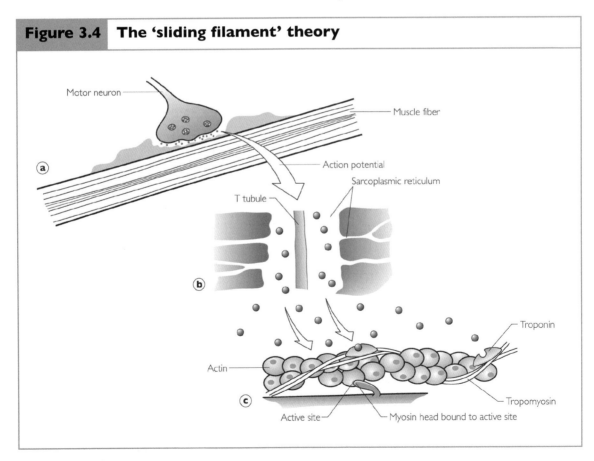

Figure 3.5 A typical motor neuron

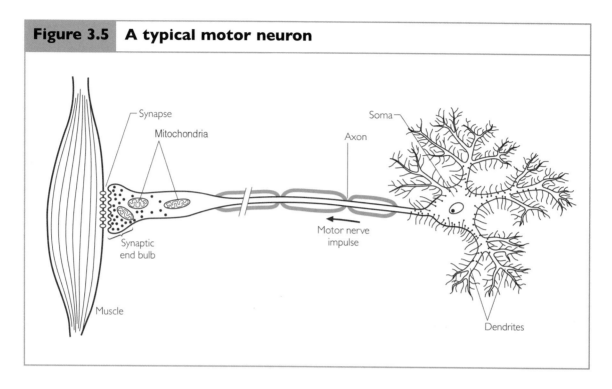

quadriceps, a motor neuron might make contact with thousands of muscle fibers. A motor neuron and the fibers it stimulates to contract are called a *motor unit*. If an action potential is sent, all of the fibers in the motor unit will contract, known as the 'all or none' principle. It is not possible to make only some of the fibers fed by the motor unit signal contract.

2. At the end of each motor neuron axon, in close proximity to the muscle fiber to be contracted, is an *axon terminal*. The axon terminal physically spreads out to become larger than the axon itself. This part is called the *synaptic end bulb* because it looks like a bulb and is next to a gap or *synapse*. When the action potential reaches the synaptic end bulb, it causes depolarization of the covering of the end bulb (the *presynaptic membrane*). Depolarization is a process in which the movement of sodium and potassium ions

(charged particles) causes an electrical current to flow. This is regulated by something known as the *sodium–potassium pump*. The depolarization process enables a neurotransmitter called *acetylcholine,* which is stored in the end bulb, to be released across the gap between the presynaptic membrane of the end bulb and the *postsynaptic membrane* (where acetylcholine is collected by the muscle) of the muscle fiber (see Figure 3.6). The motor neuron axon and the muscle fibers do not physically touch.

3. When enough acetylcholine reaches the postsynaptic membrane of the muscle fiber it can depolarize the membrane. This creates an action potential that stimulates the release of calcium from its store in the *sarcoplasmic reticulum,* which surrounds each myofibril. The calcium uncovers 'binding sites' on the actin molecules that provide a connection for the cross-bridges on the myosin molecules. The cross-bridges are like arms that pull the

Figure 3.6	Pre- and postsynaptic membranes

refers to the brief contraction of all the muscle fibers in a motor unit in response to a single electrical impulse from the brain. In slow-twitch fibers each contraction lasts for between 100 and 200 milliseconds, whereas in fast-twitch fibers the contraction lasts for under 100 milliseconds. The two broad categories of fiber differ with respect to the speed and force of the contraction and the type of fuel they use to do this.

Slow-twitch (type I) muscle fibers

Slow-twitch fibers, otherwise known as slow-oxidative, are the smallest type of fibers and are used for endurance-type activities and posture control. They have many mitochondria (see page 37) and therefore use oxygen and fat as their main fuel source for contraction. The number and size of mitochondria can be increased by endurance training, which means that more oxygen can be delivered to the muscle for the same intensity of exercise, leading to a greater energy output.

Slow-twitch fibers also have many capillaries to supply blood. These fibers are good at extracting oxygen from the blood as they contain large amounts of myoglobin, which is the oxygen carrier in the muscle. The myoglobin also gives the fibers a reddish color. As can be seen in Figure 3.7, slow-twitch fibers contract smoothly and do not generate as much force as fast-twitch fibers but are more resistant to fatigue.

actin and myosin protein molecules across each other (see also page 39).

4. *Adenosine triphosphate* (ATP) is the fuel within the body that provides the energy for the cross-bridges to pull the actin and myosin proteins (muscle fibers) together. This action is known as muscle contraction.

Each electrical signal (twitch) lasts for a very short time, so the brain needs to keep sending the signals to maintain the muscle contraction. When the brain stops sending the signals, the muscle returns to its original length.

TASK

Briefly describe how muscle contracts as if you were explaining it to someone with no knowledge of physiology.

Types of muscle fiber

Even though there are many different types of muscle fiber, they are usually grouped into two types: fast- and slow-twitch. The term 'twitch'

Fast-twitch (type II) muscle fibers

Fast-twitch (type II) fibers are powerful but are quick to fatigue. Generally, they have fewer mitochondria and therefore use glucose as their main fuel source. As the amount of myoglobin is less, they appear white in color.

Fast-twitch fibers can be split into two groups: type IIa and type IIb.

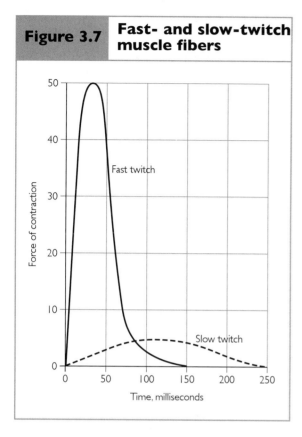

Figure 3.7 Fast- and slow-twitch muscle fibers

Type IIa fibers

Type IIa fibers are also known as fast oxidative glycolytic fibers because they can use both oxygen (aerobic) and glucose (anaerobic) as a fuel to contract (see pages 92–93). Like slow-twitch fibers, type IIa fibers contain large amounts of capillaries and myoglobin that allows them to contract aerobically but also contain stores of glycogen so that they can contract anaerobically. Type IIa fibers can produce more force than type I fibers but not as much as type IIb fibers. Similarly, the contraction speed and force generation of these fibers are greater than type I fibers but not as great as type IIb fibers. Type IIa fibers are also known as intermediate fibers because they are

between Ia and IIb fibers in terms of size. Type IIa fibers are used when type I fibers cannot cope with the workload of an exercise.

Type IIb fibers

Type IIb fibers are also known as fast glycolytic fibers as they can only use glucose as a fuel to contract (see pages 92–93). They are the most forceful and largest of the muscle fibers and are used when type I and type IIa fibers cannot cope with the workload of an exercise. Type IIb fibers have limited amounts of mitochondria and myoglobin and therefore look white in comparison with slow-twitch fibers. These fibers can generate more force than other types because the space left due to the lack of mitochondria is filled with more contractile proteins such as actin and myosin. Because the fibers are solely anaerobic, however, they are quick to fatigue compared with slow-twitch fibers.

Table 3.1 shows the common characteristics of the three groups of muscle fibers.

NEED TO KNOW

All muscles in the body contain a mixture of fast- and slow-twitch fibers. This is genetically imprinted from birth.

Fiber distribution and modification

Most skeletal muscles contain a mixture of all three types of muscle fiber, but their proportion varies depending on the usual action of the muscle. For example, postural muscles have a higher proportion of type I fibers as they are

Table 3.1	Common characteristics of muscle fiber types		
	Type I	Type IIa	Type IIb
Contraction time	Slow	Fast	Very fast
Size of motor neuron	Small	Large	Very large
Resistance to fatigue	High	Intermediate	Low
Activity used for	Aerobic	Long-term anaerobic	Short-term anaerobic
Force production	Low	High	Very high
Mitochondrial density	High	High	Low
Capillary density	High	Intermediate	Low
Oxidative capacity	High	High	Low
Glycolytic capacity	Low	High	High
Major storage fuel	Triglycerides	CP, glycogen	CP, glycogen

Key: CP = creatine phosphate

normally required to contract for long periods of time and therefore need to be resistant to fatigue. Muscles such as those of the shoulders and arms, which are not constantly active but are used intermittently to produce large amounts of tension, such as in lifting and throwing, have a higher proportion of type IIa and type IIb fibers.

Even though most skeletal muscles are a mixture of all three types of fiber, the muscle fibers in any one motor unit are all the same. In addition, the different muscle fibers within a muscle may be used in various ways, depending on need. For example, if only a weak contraction is needed in a certain muscle to perform a task, only type I fibers are activated by their motor units in that muscle. If a stronger contraction is needed, the motor units of type IIa fibers are activated in conjunction with those of type I fibers in that

muscle. If a maximal contraction is required, all motor units within that muscle are activated. Activation of the various motor units is determined in the brain and spinal cord.

Although the number of each type of muscle fiber within a particular muscle never changes, the characteristics of those present can be altered through exercise. Endurance-type exercises, such as running or swimming, result in cardiovascular and respiratory changes that mean the skeletal muscles receive better supplies of oxygen and carbohydrates. This causes a gradual adaptation in the characteristics of type IIb fibers into the characteristics of type IIa fibers. The transformed muscle fibers show a slight increase in diameter, mitochondria, blood capillaries and strength. These changes do not contribute to increased muscle mass. On the other hand, exercises that require great strength for short periods of time, such as weight lifting, produce an increase in the size and strength of type IIb fibers. However, we are what we were born with and can influence the characteristics of our muscle fibers only by a small percentage.

TASK

List and describe the common characteristics of the different types of skeletal muscle fibers.

Types of muscle contraction

Muscle contractions are classified according to what happens to the length of the muscle in the contraction.

Isotonic contractions

Isotonic contractions occur when a muscle contracts while lifting and lowering a resistance against gravity. This type of contraction can be divided into two types: *concentric* and *eccentric*. A type of contraction known as *isokinetic* (meaning same speed) is normally used only with specialized testing equipment.

Concentric contractions

A concentric contraction occurs when the muscle doing the work (the *prime mover* or *agonist*) shortens in length when contracting against a resistance. In other words, the ends of the muscle come together, for example in the lifting stage of a bicep curl when the weight is being lifted upward. When using free weights, the muscle doing the main work is always contracting concentrically when the weight is moving upward, against gravity. This is slightly

different with resistance machines (the system of pulleys means that the limb moving the weight may not be moving upward against gravity, but the weights stack will be), but the muscle doing the main work will be working concentrically when the weight stack is moving up.

Eccentric contractions

An eccentric contraction occurs when the muscle acting as the prime mover gets longer when contracting against a resistance, for example when the weight is being lowered during a bicep curl. Here the ends of the muscle are moving away from each other. In fast movements, muscles working eccentrically have a braking effect.

Isometric contractions

An isometric contraction occurs when there is no change in muscle length when contracting against a resistance, for example if a weight is lifted and then held still so that the ends of the muscle do not move either together or away from each other. From a program design point of view, it is important to be aware that isometric contractions can raise blood pressure.

TASK

Briefly describe the terms eccentric, concentric and isometric.

The roles of muscle in the body

The role of an individual muscle can change depending on the type of exercise or activity it is participating in at a specific time. These roles are normally categorized into the following groups: *agonists, antagonists, synergists* and *stabilizers*. Table 3.2 describes each role.

Agonist–antagonist pairs

Muscles are said to work in pairs across joints as they can only pull (contract) and not push. Imagine a muscle pair such as the biceps brachii and triceps brachii in the arm. When the bicep contracts with greater force, it decreases the angle of the joint (flexion), whereas the tricep stretches to allow this movement. In contrast, when the tricep contracts with greater force than the bicep, it increases the angle of the joint (extension) and the bicep stretches to allow the movement. If both muscles contracted with the same amount of force or tension, the joint angle would not move.

The muscle that contracts with the most force is called the agonist and causes the joint to move. The other muscle of the pair is called the antagonist. The amount of force produced by the antagonist can vary. Take the example of kicking a ball. The quadriceps are the agonist group as they contract to extend the knee joint. The hamstrings are the antagonist group as they try to control the speed of the extension by contracting slightly. This is known as co-contraction. The amount of co-contraction in the antagonist muscle will decrease through practice of the movement.

When strength training it is important that both agonists and antagonists are trained to create muscle balance. If either the agonist or antagonist is much stronger or less flexible than the other, the joint that is crossed by the two muscles may be pulled out of alignment to create poor posture. For example if the quadriceps are much stronger than the hamstrings, they will pull on the point of attachment at the front of the pelvis (the rectus femoris) and tilt the pelvis forward. In turn this will lead to an increase in the curvature of the lumbar spine, known as lordosis (see page 19). This is the case for muscle pairs at all joints: there are published guidelines as to typical strength ratios between the pairs (for example Norkin and White, 1995) that should be reflected in any strength training program.

Table 3.2	Roles of different muscle types
Type I	Description
Agonist	A muscle that is responsible for the main action or movement (also known as the prime mover). For example, the agonist in a shoulder press is the deltoid muscle group.
Antagonist	A muscle that directly opposes the agonist. For example, the antagonist in a shoulder press is the latissimus dorsi.
Stabilizer	A muscle that stabilizes a joint so the other muscles (agonists) are able to move the levers around the joint. For example, the transversus abdominis is a stabilizer for the pelvis.
Synergist	A muscle that helps the agonist to carry out its movement. For example, the tricep is a synergist for the bench press.

Planes of movement

Planes are a useful way of describing movements of the body. The word 'plane' is used to describe an imaginary flat surface at various angles to the body. Movement of the human body can occur in three planes: *sagittal*, *frontal* and *transverse* (see Figure 3.8).

Sagittal (or median) plane

The sagittal or median plane splits the body into left and right sides (but not necessarily equal halves). The movements distinctive to this plane are flexion and extension. Examples of resistance exercises in this plane include bicep curls or leg extensions.

Figure 3.8 **Planes of movement**

Frontal (or coronal) plane

The frontal or coronal plane divides the body into front and back sections. The movements distinctive to this plane are abduction and adduction. Examples of resistance exercises in this plane include lateral pull-downs or lateral shoulder raises.

Transverse (or horizontal) plane

The transverse or horizontal plane splits the body into upper (superior) and lower (inferior) sections. The movements distinctive to this plane are medial (internal) and lateral (external) rotation. An example of a resistance exercise in this plane is a chest press.

Exercises or movements can place various amounts of stress on joints depending on which plane of movement is used to perform the exercise. For example, the ligaments in the knee joint allow it to move in the sagittal plane but are stressed in the frontal and transverse planes. For rehabilitation purposes, exercises are often prescribed in relation to the plane of movement for a particular joint.

TASK

Choose five resistance training exercises. Name the agonist, antagonist, synergists and stabilizers for each exercise and state the plane in which the movement occurs.

Muscle and movement

As a health and fitness instructor it is useful to know the names and locations (including origins and insertions) of the major muscle groups in the body (see Figure 3.9a and 3.9b) and the movements they create when contracting. When muscles contract, they either create movement or stabilize the bones that they are attached to. There are many terms used in anatomy to describe movements of the body. It can help to remember some of these movements by linking them to specific resistance training exercises. Common terms and associated exercises are listed from page 52.

Figure 3.9

Figure 3.9 (a) Major muscle groups (front view) and (b) Major muscle groups (rear view)

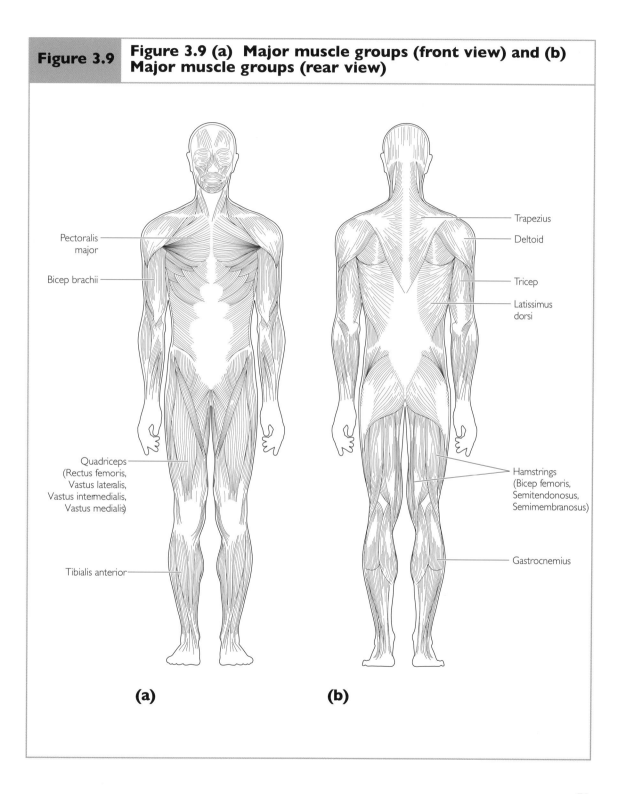

Pectoralis major

Bicep brachii

Quadriceps
(Rectus femoris,
Vastus lateralis,
Vastus intermedialis,
Vastus medialis)

Tibialis anterior

Trapezius

Deltoid

Tricep

Latissimus dorsi

Hamstrings
(Bicep femoris,
Semitendonosus,
Semimembranosus)

Gastrocnemius

(a)

(b)

Flexion

The term flexion (*flex* meaning to bend) is used when the angle between the moving bones gets smaller, for example the forearm coming toward the upper arm in a bicep curl. Another example is illustrated in Figure 3.10, where the torso is bent forward. This is known as forward flexion of the spine or trunk.

Extension

Extension (*exten* meaning to stretch) is the opposite of flexion and occurs when the joint angle gets larger. An example of this is a straight-leg movement in a backward direction in the sagittal plane, such as a hip extension. Another example is shown in Figure 3.11, where the torso is bent backward. This is known as extension of the spine or trunk.

Figure 3.10   **Forward flexion of the trunk**

Figure 3.11   **Extension of the trunk**

Hyperflexion/extension

The word hyper (meaning more than or excessive) in this sense, refers to a movement beyond the normal range of motion for a particular joint.

Lateral flexion

This refers to bending to the side. An example is shown in Figure 3.12, known as lateral flexion of the spine or trunk.

Figure 3.12 **Lateral flexion of the trunk**

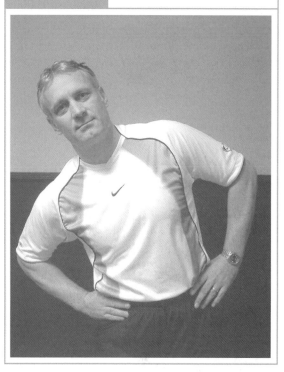

Abduction

Ab means away and *duct* means to lead, and the term abduction is used to describe a movement away from the midline of the body (see Figure 3.13a). An example is a lateral shoulder raise, where the arm moves away from the body in the frontal plane.

Figure 3.13a   Abduction

Adduction

Ad means toward, and the term adduction is used to describe a movement toward the midline of the body (see Figure 3.13b). An example of this is a lat pull-down.

Figure 3.13b   Adduction

Rotation

This term is used to describe a bone revolving around its own axis, for example rotation at the ulna-radius joint when turning the palm face down from a face-up position and vice versa. Another example is the head rotating from side to side, as if saying no (see Figures 3.14a and b).

Figure 3.14b **Rotation**

Figure 3.14a **Rotation**

Medial rotation

This term describes any inward rotational movement, for example when the upper arm (humerus) rotates toward the body (see Figure 3.15a). This is a common resistance exercise used for the muscles known as the shoulder 'rotator cuff.'

Lateral rotation

This term describes any outward rotational movement, for example when the upper arm (humerus) rotates away from the body (see Figure 3.15b). This is also a rotator cuff exercise.

Figure 3.15a Medial rotation

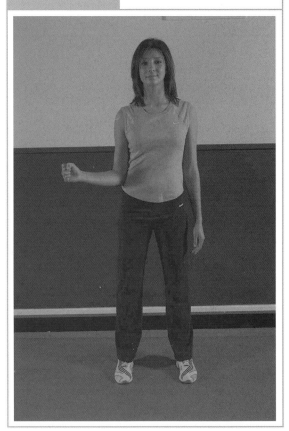

Figure 3.15b Lateral rotation

Elevation and depression

Elevation describes an upward movement of a part of the body, such as lifting the shoulders up in a shoulder shrug exercise. Depression refers to a downward movement of a part of the body, such as the shoulders going down from an elevated position. See Figures 3.16a and b.

Figure 3.16b Depression

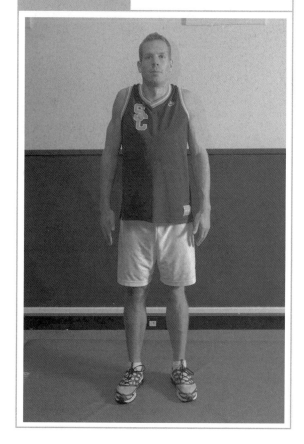

Figure 3.16a Elevation

Retraction and protraction

Retraction refers to a movement that involves drawing part of the body back, for example pulling the shoulders back from a protracted position. Protraction describes a movement that involves part of the body going forward in the transverse plane. For example, when the shoulders go forward, this is known as protraction. See Figures 3.17a and b.

Figure 3.17b **Protraction**

Figure 3.17a **Retraction**

Pronation and supination

Pronation is used to describe the palm of the hand or the sole of the foot being turned down; supination is used to describe the palm of the hand or the sole of the foot being turned up. See Figures 3.18a and b.

Figure 3.18b | **Supination**

Figure 3.18a | **Pronation**

Inversion, eversion, plantar flexion and dorsiflexion

Inversion occurs when the sole of the foot is turned inward, whereas eversion describes the foot being turned outward. Plantar flexion refers to bending the foot at the ankle joint so the foot is pointing down, whereas dorsiflexion refers to bending the foot at the ankle joint so the foot is pointing up. See Figures 3.19a–d.

| **Figure 3.19** | **(a) Inversion; (b) Eversion; (c) Plantar flexion; (d) Dorsiflexion** |

Circumduction

Circumduction is the circular movement of a part of the body, for example when doing 'windmills' with the arms. Circumduction can only occur at synovial joints (see pages 27–29).

Major muscles: their location and available movement

Individual muscles can be responsible for several movements depending on the position of the associated limbs. Tables 3.3 to 3.8 provide an overview of the locations and main movements of the major muscles.

Table 3.3	**Locations of the shoulder joint muscles**	
	Origin	Insertion
Pectoralis major	Clavicle and sternum	Proximal part of the humerus
Latissimus dorsi	Illiac crest, sacrum, lumbar and lower thoracic vertebrae	Proximal anterior part of the humerus
Deltoid	Distal third of the clavicle (anterior fibers) and whole ridge of the scapula (posterior fibers)	Lateral midpart of the humerus
Biceps brachii	Top of the scapula	Proximal part of the radius
Triceps brachii	Long head – scapula Lateral head – humerus Medial head – humerus	Olecranon of the ulna Olecranon of the ulna Olecranon of the ulna
Supraspinatus	Groove in top of the scapula	Lateral head of the humerus
Subscapularis	Underneath of the scapula	Medial head of the humerus
Infraspinatus	Flat body of the scapula	Lateral/posterior head of the humerus
Teres minor	Lateral medial wing of the scapula	Posterior head of the humerus
Teres major	Lateral inferior wing of the scapula	Medial proximal third of the humerus

Table 3.4	Movements of the muscles of the shoulder joint					
	Flexion	Extension	Abduction	Adduction	Medial rotation	Lateral rotation
Pectoralis major				×	×	
Latissimus dorsi		×		×	×	
Deltoid	x*f*	x*p*	×		x*f*	x*p*
Biceps brachii	×					
Triceps brachii		×				
Supraspinatus			×			
Subscapularis					×	
Infraspinatus				×		×
Teres minor		×		×		×
Teres major		×		x*a*	x*a*	

Key: *p* = posterior fibers; *f* = anterior fibers; *a* = assists

Table 3.5 Locations of the muscles of the hip joint

	Origin	Insertion
Hip flexors: Rectus femoris Iliopsoas	Bottom front of the pelvis Last thoracic and lumbar vertebrae and front of the pelvis	Proximal anterior part of the tibia Proximal medial part of the femur
Hip extensors: Gluteus maximus	Sacrum, coccyx and medial posterior part of the pelvis (iliac crest)	Proximal posterior third of the femur
Hamstrings: Biceps femoris Semimembranosus Semitendinosus	Ischium (all); bicep femoris also attaches to the ischium	Head of the fibula and lateral side of the tibia Proximal lateral posterior, part of the tibia
Hip adductors: Adductor brevis Adductor longus Adductor magnus Gracilis Pectineus	Pubic bone (all); gracilis also attaches to the ischium	Proximal posterior third of the femur Posterior middle part of the femur Whole posterior of the femur Proximal inside part of the tibia Proximal medial part of the femur
Hip abductors: Gluteus medius Gluteus minimus	Posterior middle part of the pelvis (gluteus minimus); the gluteus medius lies above this	Proximal lateral part of the femur (greater trochanter) for the gluteus minimus and medius
Tensor fascia latae	Posterior lateral part of the pelvis	Proximal lateral side of the tibia for the tensor fascia latae

Table 3.6	Movements of the muscles of the hip joint					
	Flexion	Extension	Abduction	Adduction	Lateral rotation	Medial rotation
Rectus femoris	×					
Iliopsoas	×				×	
Biceps femoris		×				
Semimembranosus		×				
Semitendinosus		×				
Adductor brevis	×			×		×
Adductor longus	×			×		×
Adductor magnus	×f	×p		×		×
Gracilis				×		×
Pectineus	×			×		
Gluteus maximus		×			×	
Gluteus medius			×			×
Gluteus minimus			×			×
Tensor fascia latae	×		×			

Key: f = anterior fibers, p = posterior fibers

Table 3.7	Locations of the muscles of the knee and ankle joints	
	Origin	Insertion
Quadriceps: Vastus lateralis Vastus medialis Vastus intermedius Rectus femoris	Whole of femur (lateral, medial and anterior) for all vastus (and greater trochanter for lateralis) For rectus femoris see the hip joint (page 63)	Proximal anterior part of the tibia (via patella into tibial tuberosity)
Hamstrings: Bicep femoris Semitendinosus Semimembranosus	See hip joint (page 63)	See hip joint (page 63)
Calf: Gastrocnemius Soleus Tibialis anterior	Proximal medial and lateral femur (condyles) Proximal fibula and medial tibia Proximal lateral half of the tibia	Calcaneus (through Achilles tendon) First metatarsal in the foot

TASK

Try to identify all of the major muscles in the body and list their origins, insertions and main movements.

Effects of exercise on muscle

Short-term effects

The short-term effects of exercise on muscle include the following:

1. Capillary dilation, which allows for increased blood supply.

2. Increased muscle temperature, which increases pliability (stretch) and power.
3. Increased oxygen demand and use by muscles being used in order to supply the increased number of fibers being used.
4. Muscle fibers contract at a faster rate due to increased nerve stimulation. The contracting muscle fibers, which squeeze the walls of blood vessels, push blood further along the vessels in a type of pump action known as the 'muscle pump.'

Long-term effects

The long-term effects of exercise on muscle include the following:

1. Improved muscle tone.
2. Improved posture.

Table 3.8	Movements of the muscles of the knee and ankle joints				
	Knee flexion	Knee extension	Plantar flexion	Dorsiflexion	Inversion
Vastus lateralis		✕			
Vastus medialis		✕			
Vastus intermedius		✕			
Rectus femoris		✕			
Bicep femoris	✕				
Semitendinosus	✕				
Semimembranosus	✕				
Gastrocnemius	✕		✕		
Soleus			✕		
Tibialis anterior			✕		✕

3. Increase in muscle bulk (hypertrophy) and strength. This is due to an increase in the number of contractile proteins (actin and myosin), an increase in the number and size of myofibrils per muscle fiber and increased amounts of connective, tendinous and ligamentous tissues.

4. Increased numbers of enzymes and stored nutrients.

5. Increased number of capillaries and mitochondria in slow-twitch fibers.

EXAMPLE QUESTIONS

3.1 What is the main fuel of slow-twitch fibers?

a) fat and oxygen
b) protein
c) glucose
d) creatine phosphate

3.2 What is the main fuel of fast-twitch fibers?

a) fat and oxygen
b) protein
c) glucose
d) alcohol

3.3 Which type of muscle can be found in arteries?

a) striated
b) cardiac
c) skeletal
d) smooth

3.4 Which type of muscle can be found in the heart?

a) striated
b) cardiac
c) skeletal
d) smooth

3.5 In muscle contraction, which neurotransmitter stimulates the release of calcium?

a) adenosine triphosphate
b) acetylcholine
c) actin
d) myosin

EXAMPLE QUESTIONS cont.

3.6 What is the name for the type of contraction when the muscle lengthens?

a) isometric

b) concentric

c) eccentric

d) isokinetic

3.7 What is the name for the type of contraction when the muscle shortens?

a) isometric

b) concentric

c) eccentric

d) isokinetic

3.8 What is the name for a muscle that opposes the prime mover?

a) agonist

b) stabilizer

c) synergist

d) antagonist

3.9 What is the name for a muscle that assists the prime mover?

a) agonist

b) stabilizer

c) synergist

d) antagonist

3.10 What is the name for a muscle that performs the main action?

a) agonist

b) stabilizer

c) synergist

d) antagonist

EXAMPLE QUESTIONS cont.

3.11 Which movements are associated with the sagittal plane?
   a) inversion and eversion
   b) adduction and abduction
   c) pronation and supination
   d) flexion and extension

3.12 What is the name of the movement of the foot when the toes point down?
   a) inversion
   b) eversion
   c) plantar flexion
   d) dorsiflexion

Further reading

Abrahams, P., Craven, J. and Lumley, J. (2005) *Illustrated Clinical Anatomy*, Hodder Arnold

Baechle, R.T. (2000) *Essentials of Strength Training and Conditioning* (2nd ed.), Human Kinetics

Marieb, E.N. (2001) *Human Anatomy and Physiology*, Benjamin Cummings

Norkin, C.C. and White, D.J. (1995) *Measurement of Joint Motion: A guide to goniometry*, F.A. Davis

Porter, S. (2002) *The Anatomy Workbook*, Butterworth Heinemann

Sewell, D., Watkins, P. and Griffin, M. (2005) *Sport and Exercise Science: An Introduction*, Hodder Arnold

Tortora, G.J. and Grabowski, S.R. (2003) *Principles of Anatomy and Physiology* (10th ed.), Wiley

Wilson, K.J.W. and Waugh, A. (1998) *Ross and Wilson Anatomy and Physiology in Health and Illness*, Churchill Livingstone

NOTES

CARTILAGE, LIGAMENTS AND TENDONS

4

OBJECTIVES

After completing this chapter, you will be able to

1 Describe the structure and function of cartilage.

2 List and describe the different types of cartilage and give examples of each.

3 Describe the structure and function of ligaments.

4 Describe the structure and function of tendons.

Instructing Physical Activity and Exercise Knowledge

Anatomy

- Articulations and joint movements.

- Structure and movement potential/anatomic limitations of major joints (shoulder, hip, knee, elbow).

- Muscle attachment sites.

- Stability vs movement within each type of joint.

- Ligaments; articular cartilage.

Introduction

This chapter deals with connective tissue within the human body, in particular cartilage, ligament and tendon, from a perspective of structure, function and the effects of exercise. Instructors should be able to list the types and roles of cartilage and ligament in the human body.

Later chapters provide physiologic and biomechanical principles that, together with the anatomic knowledge covered in this chapter, provide the instructor with the understanding and ability to design appropriate exercise programs for apparently healthy individuals and to understand the effects of various types of exercise on the human body.

Cartilage

Structure, function and types

Cartilage is a dense, tough connective tissue that forms only a very small portion of the adult skeleton. It consists of a mixture of

- Calcaneofibular – between the calcaneus and the fibula
- Anterior and posterior talofibular – between the talus and the fibula.

Between them, the deltoid and lateral collateral ligaments allow the foot to move in flexion and extension but provide stability in lateral movements such as inversion and eversion. In other words, they prevent the ankle from rolling in or out. See Figure 4.3.

Figure 4.3	**Common ligaments of the ankle**

NEED TO KNOW

It was a cruciate ligament injury that prevented Michael Owen from taking any further part in the 2006 World Cup Finals.

Tendons

Structure and function

Tendons are bluish white, slightly elastic fascia tissues that connect muscles to bone. Tendons are made up of the sheaths that surround the muscle fibers and attach to the periosteum covering on the bone. In some cases the area of connection is relatively small, for example the biceps brachii tendons, but in other cases the tendon can be spread out in sheets over a wide area, such as the tibialis anterior. The latter type of tendon attachments are called *aponeuroses*.

When muscles contract they pull from the middle and therefore exert a pulling force on the tendons at each end of the muscle. As the tendons are connected to bone, they will attempt to pull the bones together. If one of the bones remains in a fixed position, the other bone will move toward it and create movement.

Tendons stretch only slightly, and not as much as muscle tissue, and prolonged tension on tendon tissue may result in tearing. Tendons are reasonably slow to heal as their blood supply is less than that of muscles. As with ligaments, tendons will become stronger with weight-bearing activity.

In the case of extreme force, it is also possible for the tendon to pull away from the attachment point at the periosteum. This is called an *avulsion*. This can be a partial tear, where there is still some tendon attached, or a complete rupture, where the entire tendon is torn from the periosteum. If a complete rupture occurs, the muscle will have no attachment at one end and will therefore be unable to move the bone it is attached to. This requires surgery, whereas a partial tear can heal in time. Tendons can also become inflamed through repetitive use. This type of injury is known as tendonitis (*itis* meaning inflammation).

TASK

Describe the structure and function of cartilage (all types), ligament and tendon tissue.

The effects of exercise on cartilage, ligament and tendon

Short-term effects

During exercise, there will be an increased blood supply to both ligaments and tendons. As a result, heat will be produced, which makes these structures slightly more elastic and less susceptible to injury.

Long-term effects

Both ligaments and tendons are capable of becoming stronger after a long-term period of regular exercise, in particular resistance training. Ligaments can actually hypertrophy (grow in size) by a small amount.

EXAMPLE QUESTIONS

4.1 What type of cartilage covers the end of a bone?

a) fibro
b) elastic
c) articular
d) tendinous

4.2 What type of cartilage can be found in the nose and ear?

a) fibro
b) elastic
c) articular
d) tendinous

4.3 What type of cartilage can be found between vertebral bodies?

a) fibro
b) elastic
c) articular
d) tendinous

4.4 What color is articular cartilage?

a) blue
b) bluey-white
c) white
d) grayish white

4.5 What is the main function of articular cartilage?

a) shock absorption
b) support
c) prevent friction
d) release synovial fluid

EXAMPLE QUESTIONS cont.

4.6 What type of cartilage gets lubricated by synovial fluid?

a) fibro

b) elastic

c) articular

d) tendinous

4.7 What is the main function of fibro cartilage?

a) shock absorption

b) support

c) prevent friction

d) release synovial fluid

4.8 What is the main function of elastic cartilage?

a) shock absorption

b) support

c) prevent friction

d) release synovial fluid

4.9 Which type of tissue connects bone to bone?

a) cartilage

b) tendon

c) ligament

d) muscle

4.10 Which type of tissue connects muscle to bone?

a) cartilage

b) tendon

c) ligament

d) muscle

EXAMPLE QUESTIONS cont.

4.11 What is the name of the fibro cartilage in the knee joint?
a) collateral
b) periosteum
c) intervertebral
d) meniscus

4.12 Which type of tissue does the statement 'allows wanted but prevents unwanted movement' relate to?
a) cartilage
b) tendon
c) ligament
d) muscle

Further reading

Abrahams, P., Craven, J. and Lumley, J. (2005) *Illustrated Clinical Anatomy*, Hodder Arnold

Baechle, R.T. (1994) *Essentials of Strength Training and Conditioning*, Human Kinetics

Porter, S. (2002) *The Anatomy Workbook*, Butterworth Heinemann

Sewell, D., Watkins, P. and Griffin, M. (2005) *Sport and Exercise Science: An Introduction*, Hodder Arnold

Tortora, G.J. and Grabowski, S.R. (2003) *Principles of Anatomy and Physiology* (10th ed.), Wiley

Wilson, K.J.W. and Waugh, A. (1998) *Ross and Wilson Anatomy and Physiology in Health and Illness*, Churchill Livingstone

NOTES

THE NERVOUS AND ENDOCRINE SYSTEMS

5

OBJECTIVES

After completing this chapter, you will be able to

1   Describe the structure and function of the nervous system.

2   Describe the structure and function of the endocrine system.

3   Describe the roles of sensory receptors in the body.

4   Explain the roles of the autonomic and somatic branches of the peripheral nervous system.

5   Explain the roles of the sympathetic and parasympathetic branches of the autonomic nervous system.

6   List the glands and associated hormones of the endocrine system.

7   Describe the role of hormones within the endocrine system.

Instructing Physical Activity and Exercise Knowledge

Anatomy: Nervous and Endocrine Systems

- Role of the nervous system:
  - Sensory input
  - Interpretation
  - Major output

- Two parts of the nervous system:
  - Central
  - Peripheral – autonomic and somatic

- How regular activity can enhance neuromuscular connections and improve motor fitness

- Endocrine glands and associated hormones involved in exercise preparation and performance:
  - Pancreas – regulation of blood glucose
  - Adrenal glands – adrenaline

- Testosterone

Introduction

This chapter deals with the nervous and endocrine systems within the human body from a perspective of structure, function and the effects of exercise. Instructors should be able to explain and describe how both systems work within the human body.

Later chapters provide physiologic and biomechanical principles that, together with the anatomic knowledge covered in this chapter, provide the instructor with the understanding and ability to design appropriate exercise programs for apparently healthy individuals and to understand the effects of various types of exercise on the human body.

Overview of the nervous and endocrine systems

Although the nervous system and the endocrine system are separate, they work in conjunction with each other to monitor and regulate all of the systems within the body, including temperature, blood pressure, blood glucose and blood calcium. When the nervous and the endocrine systems work optimally to keep all of the other systems within limits, the body is said to be in *homeostasis*.

The main difference between the two systems is in the way they operate. The nervous system operates as a network of connecting nerve fibers that rapidly transmit electrical signals, whereas the endocrine system operates more slowly using chemical messengers called *hormones* that are secreted into the bloodstream from groups of cells known as *glands*. It is worth noting that when these hormone messengers are released from nerve endings as opposed to glands, they are known as *neurotransmitters*.

Both the nervous and the endocrine systems work on a 'lock and key' basis: the messengers (neurotransmitters and gland hormones) act as keys, and the places they deliver messages to are called locks (or *receptor cells*). Messages will only be accepted by locks if they are the correct keys: in other words, specific neurotransmitters and hormones can deliver messages only to specific sites. If the specific key is not available, there will be no effect on the lock. Take, for example, beta-blockers (commonly prescribed medication for heart conditions). If beta receptor cells combine with beta keys, the resulting message stimulates an increase in heart rate. In the case of cardiac patients, where limiting the heart rate is a necessity, chemicals that block the beta receptor cells, and thus prevent an increase in heart rate, are prescribed. These are called beta-blockers for obvious reasons.

NEED TO KNOW

It was once thought that nerve damage could never be repaired, but scientists have had recent success with regeneration of nerve tissue.

The nervous system

The nervous system has many functions in the body, for example being responsible for our perceptions, memories and behavior, as well as being responsible for muscle contraction.

Structure of the nervous system

The nervous system is divided into two parts: the central nervous system (CNS) and the peripheral nervous system (PNS). The CNS is made up of the brain, the brainstem and the spinal cord (see Figure 5.1).

The PNS is made up of a series of nerve branches that either lead into or away from the CNS. Nerves that lead away from the CNS are called *motor* or *efferent* nerves as they carry information to muscles and organs to effect a response. Nerves that lead into the CNS are called *sensory* or *afferent* nerves as they carry information back to the CNS about changes in the body.

Nerves that lead into the CNS come from groups of specialized cells around the body called *sensory receptors*. As the name implies, sensory receptors are capable of detecting changes in the body such as temperature, sight, hearing, taste and smell. Table 5.1 lists some receptors and their functions in the body.

TASK

List the common sensory receptors in the human body and give a brief description of what each one does.

When the body is in homeostasis, the sensory receptors do not relay information to the brain. If any changes are detected by the receptors away from homeostasis, information is then relayed to the brain via the sensory or afferent nerves so the brain can initiate a response. For example, if proprioceptors in the ankle ligaments detect that they are being stretched too far, the brain will respond by sending an electrical signal via the motor or efferent nerves to specific leg muscles in order to balance and stabilize the ankle.

Table 5.1	Description of sensory receptors
Receptor	Description
Proprioceptors	These are found in tissue such as muscle, tendon and joints and provide information relating to position. These receptors can be damaged easily in injuries such as ankle sprains. If this occurs, balance can be affected because of a lack of position information being relayed to the brain.
Baroreceptors	This type of receptor is mainly found in the walls of blood vessels in order to relay information to the brain regarding blood pressure.
Chemoreceptors	These receptors monitor the concentration of certain chemicals in the body, such as blood glucose level.
Thermoreceptors	These are present in all tissues of the body to detect changes in temperature.
Nociceptors	These are present in all tissues of the body and detect pain (tissue damage).

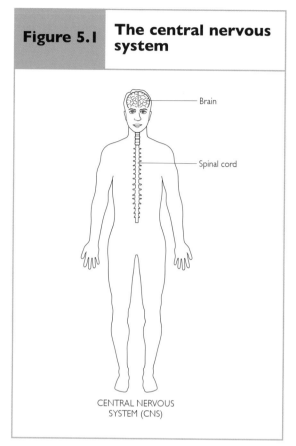

Figure 5.1 | **The central nervous system**

Brain

Spinal cord

CENTRAL NERVOUS
SYSTEM (CNS)

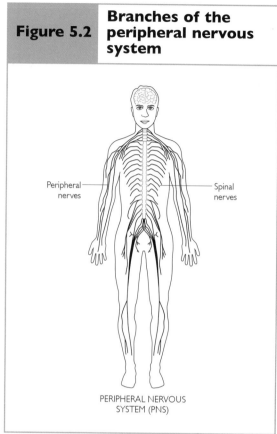

Figure 5.2 | **Branches of the peripheral nervous system**

Peripheral nerves

Spinal nerves

PERIPHERAL NERVOUS
SYSTEM (PNS)

Branches of the peripheral nervous system

The PNS has two branches, known as the *somatic branch* and the *autonomic branch*. The autonomic branch is then further subdivided into two branches, called the *sympathetic* and *parasympathetic* branches (see Figure 5.2).

In simple terms, the somatic nervous system controls voluntary actions such as moving away from danger or foul smells, whereas the autonomic nervous system controls involuntary actions such as heart rate and blood pressure.

Sympathetic nervous system

This branch of the nervous system acts almost like a stimulus to increase specific activity or stimulate specific processes in the body. Sympathetic nerves do this by releasing the neurotransmitters *adrenaline* and *noradrenaline* (as discussed on page 81, these are hormones but are called neurotransmitters as they are not secreted from glands). These neurotransmitters speed up processes in the body. For instance, adrenaline stimulates the breakdown of fat and glycogen to be used for energy production.

Parasympathetic nervous system

This branch of the nervous system has the opposite effect to that of the sympathetic nervous system: its main roles are reducing the activity of processes within the body and conserving fuel stores. The main neurotransmitter used in this system is acetylcholine, which is used in the process of muscle contraction (see pages 42–44).

TASK

Draw a diagram of the structure of the PNS, including all the branches.

The endocrine system

As discussed above, the nervous system sends messages (information) around the body by using neurotransmitters, which are hormones secreted by nerve endings. The endocrine system is another messenger system for the body that sends messages using hormones secreted by glands. This is normally done in conjunction with the nervous system: if the homeostasis of the body is disturbed, the nervous system recognizes this and in turn stimulates specific glands in the body to release hormones, which return the body to homeostasis. Most hormones are circulated via the bloodstream, so the endocrine system can be quite slow compared with the nervous system.

The main endocrine glands include the pineal, pituitary, thyroid, parathyroid and adrenal glands (see Figure 5.3). The pineal and pituitary glands are located in the brain, whereas the other glands and tissues are located around the body. There are other tissues in the body that secrete hormones, such as the hypothalamus, pancreas, thymus, ovaries, testes, kidneys and stomach, but these are not referred to as endocrine glands.

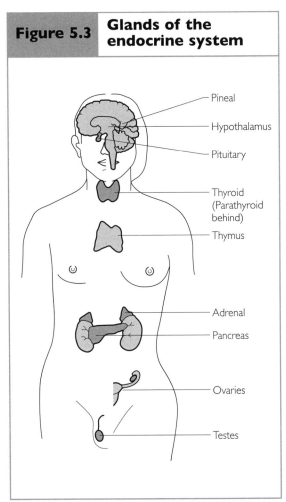

Figure 5.3 Glands of the endocrine system

NEED TO KNOW

Seasonal affective disorder (SAD), which is mainly related to the hormone melatonin, affects about 25 percent of the population.

TASK

List the common glands and tissues in the body and the hormones that they secrete.

Types of hormones

There are two main groups of hormones: lipid-soluble and water-soluble.

Lipid-soluble hormones

One common type of lipid-soluble hormone is *steroid* hormones. Cortisol, testosterone and estrogen (among others) belong to this group. Steroid hormones take a reasonable amount of time to have an effect, but their effect is usually long lasting. The main functions of this group are related to either growth function or the control of cycles in the body such as the menstruation cycle.

Water-soluble hormones

One common type of water-soluble hormones is *peptide* hormones. Examples include insulin and glucagon, which are used to control blood sugar levels. The main role of this group of hormones is to act on metabolism.

EXAMPLE QUESTIONS

5.1 Chemical messengers called hormones are secreted into the bloodstream from groups of cells known as what?

a) nerve endings

b) neurotransmitters

c) glands

d) sensory receptors

5.2 Where are neurotransmitters secreted from?

a) nerve endings

b) glands

c) axons

d) organs

5.3 What do the the brain, the brainstem and the spinal cord make up?

a) peripheral nervous system

b) central nervous system

c) somatic nervous system

d) autonomic nervous system

5.4 What is the series of nerve branches that lead into and away from the CNS known as?

a) peripheral nervous system

b) central nervous system

c) somatic nervous system

d) autonomic nervous system

5.5 Which of the following receptors sense position?

a) proprioceptors

b) chemoreceptors

c) nociceptors

d) thermoreceptors

EXAMPLE QUESTIONS cont.

5.6 Which of the following receptors sense pain?

a) proprioceptors
b) chemoreceptors
c) nociceptors
d) thermoreceptors

5.7 Which of the following receptors sense temperature?

a) proprioceptors
b) chemoreceptors
c) nociceptors
d) thermoreceptors

5.8 Which of the following receptors sense chemical composition?

a) proprioceptors
b) chemoreceptors
c) nociceptors
d) thermoreceptors

5.9 Cortisol and noradrenaline are secreted by which gland?

a) pituitary
b) parathyroid
c) pancreas
d) adrenals

5.10 Blood calcium levels are regulated by which gland?

a) pituitary
b) parathyroid
c) pancreas
d) adrenals

EXAMPLE QUESTIONS cont.

5.11 Insulin is secreted by which gland?

  a) pituitary

  b) parathyroid

  c) pancreas

  d) adrenals

5.12 Cortisol, testosterone and estrogen belong to a group of hormones known as what?

  a) peptide hormones

  b) pancreatic hormones

  c) metabolic hormones

  d) steroid hormones

Further reading

Abrahams, P., Craven, J. and Lumley, J. (2005) *Illustrated Clinical Anatomy*, Hodder Arnold

Baechle, R.T. (2000) *Essentials of Strength Training and Conditioning* (2nd ed.), Human Kinetics

Porter, S. (2002) *The Anatomy Workbook*, Butterworth Heinemann

Sewell, D., Watkins, P. and Griffin, M. (2005) *Sport and Exercise Science: An Introduction*, Hodder Arnold

Tortora, G.J. and Grabowski, S.R. (2003) *Principles of Anatomy and Physiology* (10th ed.), Wiley

Wilson, K.J.W. and Waugh, A. (1998) *Ross and Wilson Anatomy and Physiology in Health and Illness*, Churchill Livingstone

NOTES

ENERGY SYSTEMS

6

OBJECTIVES

After completing this chapter, you will be able to

1 Name and describe the structure of adenosine triphosphate (ATP) used for muscle contraction.

2 Name and describe each system within the body that can produce ATP.

3 Explain how each energy-producing system is contributing at low, medium and high exercise intensities.

4 Name the by-products of each energy-producing system.

5 Explain the problems associated with lactic acid.

6 Suggest ways to prevent depletion of glucose stores in the body.

7 Name typical activities associated with each energy-producing system as the main contributing system.

8 Explain how fitness levels can affect the energy-producing systems being used.

Instructing Exercise and Fitness Knowledge

Basic Anatomy and Physiology
- The aerobic and anaerobic energy systems and the energy requirements of physical activity.

Instructing Physical Activity and Exercise Knowledge

Energy Systems
- ATP

- Three energy systems:
  - Creatine phosphate, anaerobic, aerobic
  - Interaction of the energy systems during a range of exercises/activities
  - Capacity of the three energy systems and adaptations in relation to training modalities
  - Effects of exercise intensity, duration and fitness levels on the energy systems used

- Use of energy nutrients at different intensities and amount of energy nutrients used at different intensities

Introduction

This chapter deals with the supply of fuel to the muscles of the body, known as 'energy systems,' and in particular the interaction of the various systems during rest and during different intensities of exercise. Instructors should be able to describe each of the different systems as well as describe how these interact during rest and exercise.

This chapter provides the instructor with the understanding of how energy systems work, which will provide the underpinning knowledge to assist in the design of appropriate exercise programs for apparently healthy individuals and in understanding the effects of various types of exercise on the human body.

Energy systems for muscular contraction

Whether the body is at rest or moving during exercise, energy must be supplied either to living systems for chemical reactions to take place or to the muscles for movement to occur. The unit of energy that is used in the body for muscles to contract is called *adenosine triphosphate* (ATP), which is sometimes known as the *energy currency* in the body.

An ATP molecule is made up of the adenosine part (a molecule of adenine and a molecule of ribose) with three (*tri* meaning three) phosphate groups bonded to each other (see Figure 6.1).

Figure 6.1 An ATP molecule

The bonds keeping the phosphates together are known as *high-energy bonds*. If one of the phosphates is split from the adenosine molecule, a large amount of energy is released to be used for muscle contraction (see Figure 6.2). Heat is also given off when a phosphate splits from the adenosine. This leaves an adenosine molecule with only two phosphates, which is called *adenosine diphosphate* or *ADP* (*di* meaning two).

Figure 6.2 Phosphate splitting from an ATP molecule

= Energy release from ATP

The main problem with this is that there is only enough ATP in the body to last for about four seconds, so a phosphate must be reattached to the ADP to make ATP in order for the process to start again. This is called *resynthesis*. Carbohydrates, fats and proteins are digested to provide a source of phosphate.

This process of resynthesis occurs on a continuous basis in the body, but the amount of energy in the form of ATP that is needed depends on the amount of muscle contraction or exercise being carried out: obviously, when exercising at a higher level, more ATP is needed to supply the energy. The place in the muscle where the ATP is used to provide energy for muscle contraction is called the *mitochondria* or the 'powerhouse.'

Carbohydrates are used to supply energy in the form of ATP mainly in the short term, and fats are used mainly in the long term. Protein is usually used only as a standby source of ATP energy. There are three systems within the body that supply the energy from the digested food to the muscles that need it: the creatine phosphate (ATP–CP) system, the *aerobic* system and the *anaerobic* system.

The creatine phosphate system (ATP–CP)

This system is also known as the PCr or phosphocreatine system. As ATP stores last only for a few seconds, the body needs a system that can resynthesize ADP to ATP very quickly when an individual starts to exercise. The ATP–CP system can do this almost immediately, but the body contains only a very short-term supply. As a result, the system can be used for up to about 10 seconds only but can be used over and over again as long as a recovery period of about three minutes is allowed (this recovery period can be low-intensity exercise). Once the creatine phosphate molecule has given its phosphate to the ADP, which in turn becomes ATP, a phosphate can be broken off to release energy (see Figure 6.3).

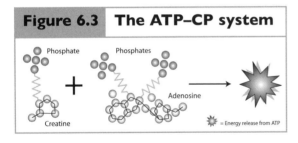

Figure 6.3 The ATP–CP system

Phosphate   Phosphates

Adenosine

Creatine   ✷ = Energy release from ATP

This system is very simple and produces no waste products. However, it is not very efficient: for every one molecule of creatine phosphate used, only one molecule of ATP is produced. After the store of creatine phosphate in the body has been used, the body must switch to another system to supply phosphate in order to resynthesize ADP. Imagine this system in terms of driving a car. The ATP–CP system is the first system to be used in the body, just like first gear is the first gear to be

used in a car. If you were to drive a long distance in first gear, the amount of fuel used would be enormous and therefore not very efficient. This is the same in the body: if you used only creatine phosphate as an energy source, it would run out very quickly. The body needs to move into another system to provide energy, just like the car needs to move into second gear. However, it must be noted that all energy systems are active at the same time (see page 94).

The anaerobic or lactic acid system

Glucose (without oxygen)

Glucose is a sugar found in carbohydrate foods such as potatoes, vegetables, rice, bread and fruit. When carbohydrates are digested they release glucose, which is then stored in the body as *glycogen*. Glucose in the blood and glycogen from stores in the body are then used to supply phosphates. The process of breaking down glucose to provide energy is called *anaerobic glycolysis*.

If the exercise intensity is high, this energy supply system can be maintained continuously only for two to three minutes as it produces a substance called *lactic acid* as a waste product (see Figure 6.4). Lactic acid can stop muscle contraction if too much is produced, and the greater the intensity of exercise, the more lactic acid is produced.

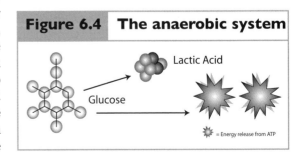

Figure 6.4 The anaerobic system

Lactic Acid

Glucose

✷ = Energy release from ATP

As this is the next system that the body uses to supply energy after the ATP–CP system, it is equivalent to using second gear in a car. If you were going on a long journey in a car, you would again use a lot of fuel if you stayed in this gear for the entire journey. It is the same in the body: only two ATP molecules are produced from each glucose molecule, so the body needs to move on to the next, more efficient system or gear.

The aerobic system

Glucose (with oxygen)

After a few minutes of exercise, oxygen is transported to the muscles to be used with glucose to provide energy in a system called *aerobic glycolysis.* As long as the intensity is not too high, and oxygen is present, there will be no build-up of lactic acid. Carbon dioxide and water are given off as waste products (see Figure 6.5).

Figure 6.5	The aerobic system using glucose

Glucose + Oxygen → $CO_2 + H_2O$
= Energy release from ATP

When oxygen is used in resynthesis it is more efficient as 38 molecules of ATP are produced per molecule of oxygen. However, one of the problems with this system is that there is only sufficient glycogen stored in the body for medium-intensity exercise of about two hours duration, if the storage is full prior to the exercise: if glycogen stores have been used up in previous exercise and have not yet been replaced, the possible duration of exercise using this system will be less. This is similar to going on a long journey in a car and having a less than full fuel tank – either you cannot travel as far or you need to refuel. Carbohydrate drinks can be taken during exercise to supply glucose to the muscles; this also spares the stores in the body. It is also important to eat a carbohydrate snack as soon as possible after exercise to replace glucose that has been used during the exercise. However, rather than rely on this system for energy, the body has another system that is even more efficient and uses fat, among other things, as a fuel.

Fat (with oxygen)

After several minutes of exercise (this time varies with fitness levels) intramuscular fat or fat that is transported to the muscle can be used in the energy process. In order for this to happen, small amounts of glucose and oxygen must be available. The place in the muscle where energy is released by breaking down fat, carbohydrate and oxygen is called the *mitochondria* (see also page 91). There is no build-up of lactic acid, but carbon dioxide, water and heat are given off as by-products (see Figure 6.6). This system is used when the exercise is of low-to-moderate intensity, such as walking or comfortable jogging. As this system uses a small amount of glucose, the exercise can be maintained only as long as glucose is available, usually about two hours (less if the exercise was started on low stores of glucose), unless carbohydrates are taken in during the exercise. **Note:** There are other ways to metabolize fat which are beyond the scope of this book.

Figure 6.6	The aerobic system using fat

Fat + Oxygen → $CO_2 + H_2O$
= Energy release from ATP

Depending on the type of fat used in this system (there are several types of fat available from food), more than 200 ATP molecules can be produced from each molecule of fat, glucose and oxygen. This makes this system very efficient in producing energy for muscle contraction. However, if stores of glucose do run out, it can be difficult for the body to break down fat. This is another reason why carbohydrate foods are important when exercising.

A person who exercises on a regular basis will move through the systems, like the gears in a car, to get to the system using fat more quickly than a person who is not used to exercise. This is simply because the body responds to the exercise regularity by becoming more efficient.

Interaction of energy systems

The body actually uses all of the above systems at the same time; however, the intensity of the exercise dictates which energy system will be used to supply the majority of the energy (see Figure 6.7).

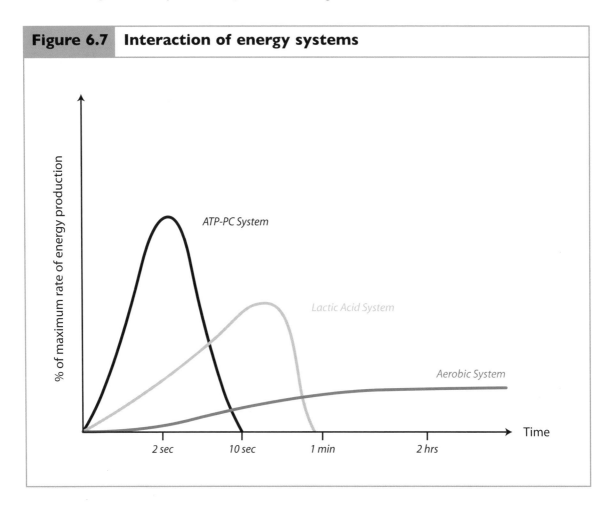

Figure 6.7   Interaction of energy systems

For example, at the start of exercise (warm-up) the demand for oxygen cannot be met quickly by the aerobic system, so the anaerobic system must contribute more to energy production. However, as the warm-up continues the capillaries in the lungs and muscles dilate, increasing the flow of oxygen so that the contribution from the aerobic systems increases. After a period of time, which in some cases can be up to 30 minutes or more (at low to medium intensity), most of the energy is provided by the fat system, with the other systems providing a small amount. If, during low- to medium-intensity exercise, the individual decides to increase to a high intensity, the sudden requirement for extra energy usually comes from extra glucose in the body.

However, the problem here is that large amounts of glucose will be needed to provide the large amount of energy required to sustain the high-intensity exercise. This means that large amounts of the by-product lactic acid will be produced, which will eventually stop the muscle from contracting. High-intensity exercise producing large amounts of lactic acid is normally only sustainable for about two minutes, and much less in unfit people.

Table 6.1 shows the main energy systems used in typical sporting activities.

Table 6.1	Major energy systems used in typical activities	
Major energy system	Performance time	Typical activities
ATP–CP	<10 seconds	Shot put 100 m sprints
Anaerobic glycolysis	20–90 seconds	200–400 m sprints Speed skating 100 m swim
Aerobic glycolysis	90 seconds to several minutes	Gymnastics 800 m run Boxing round
Fat	More than several minutes	Jogging

EXAMPLE QUESTIONS

6.1 When a phosphate molecule is reattached to ADP to make ATP, what is the process called?

a) replenishment

b) reattachment

c) regeneration

d) resynthesis

6.2 The 'powerhouse' within a muscle cell where ATP is generated aerobically is known as the what?

a) organelle

b) mitochondria

c) sarcoplasmic reticulum

d) spindle

6.3 What is anaerobic glycolysis?

a) breaking down glucose in the presence of oxygen

b) breaking down glucose without the presence of oxygen

c) converting glucose to glycogen in the presence of oxygen

d) converting glucose to glycogen without the presence of oxygen

6.4 What is aerobic glycolysis?

a) breaking down glucose in the presence of oxygen

b) breaking down glucose without the presence of oxygen

c) converting glucose to glycogen in the presence of oxygen

d) converting glucose to glycogen without the presence of oxygen

6.5 Which of the following is given off as a by-product of aerobic glycolysis?

a) ATP

b) hydrogen

c) lactic acid

d) carbon dioxide and water

EXAMPLE QUESTIONS cont.

6.6 Which of the following is given off as a by-product of anaerobic glycolysis?
a) ATP
b) hydrogen
c) lactic acid
d) carbon dioxide and water

6.7 Which of the following is produced as a result of the incomplete breakdown of fat due to a lack of available carbohydrate?
a) lactic acid
b) hydrogen
c) ketones
d) carbon dioxide and water

6.8 Which energy system contributes the most (in percentage terms) at the start of exercise?
a) anaerobic glycolysis
b) aerobic glycolysis
c) ATP–CP
d) aerobic fat

6.9 Which energy system contributes the least (in percentage terms) at the start of exercise?
a) anaerobic glycolysis
b) aerobic glycolysis
c) ATP–CP
d) aerobic (fat)

6.10 Which energy system contributes the most (in percentage terms) in short-sprint events such as the 100 meters?
a) anaerobic glycolysis
b) aerobic glycolysis
c) ATP–CP
d) aerobic (fat)

EXAMPLE QUESTIONS cont.

6.11 Which energy system contributes the most (in percentage terms) in events such as the 800 meters?

a) they are all the same

b) aerobic glycolysis

c) ATP–CP

d) lactic acid

6.12 Which energy system contributes the most (in percentage terms) in events such as jogging?

a) they are all the same

b) aerobic (fat)

c) ATP–CP

d) lactic acid

Further reading

Abrahams, P., Craven, J. and Lumley, J. (2005) *Illustrated Clinical Anatomy*, Hodder Arnold

Baechle, R.T. (2000) *Essentials of Strength Training and Conditioning*, (2nd ed.), Human Kinetics

Porter, S. (2002) *The Anatomy Workbook*, Butterworth Heinemann

Sewell, D., Watkins, P. and Griffin, M. (2005) *Sport and Exercise Science: An Introduction*, Hodder Arnold

Tortora, G.J. and Grabowski, S.R. (2003) *Principles of Anatomy and Physiology* (10th ed.), Wiley

Wilson, K.J.W. and Waugh, A. (1998) *Ross and Wilson Anatomy and Physiology in Health and Illness*, Churchill Livingstone

NOTES

THE HEART AND THE CIRCULATORY SYSTEM

OBJECTIVES

After completing this chapter, you will be able to

1 Describe the structure of the heart in relation to the layers of muscle and surrounding sheath.

2 Name and describe the sections within the heart.

3 Explain the process of heart contraction (cardiac cycle).

4 Describe the flow of blood into and away from the heart and describe the features of the associated vessels.

5 Describe the composition of blood.

6 Explain the mechanisms of venous return.

7 Explain the terms *hypertension* and *hypotension* in relation to blood pressure and how exercise affects blood pressure.

Instructing Exercise and Fitness Knowledge

Basic Anatomy and Physiology
- The location and function of the heart; the function of arteries, veins and capillaries.
- The short- and long-term effects of exercise on the heart and circulatory system.

Instructing Physical Activity and Exercise Knowledge

Anatomy: Cardiovascular System
- Anatomy of the heart:
  - The four chambers
  - Valves and control of blood flow
  - The cardiac cycle
  - Conduction systems (autonomic and intrinsic)
  - Cardiac output (regulation of stroke volume and heart rate)
  - Cardiac circulation
- Structure, function and characteristics of arteries, arterioles, veins and capillaries
- Coronary circulation

- Systemic circulation
- Pathway of oxygen from inhaled air to muscle
- Pathway of carbon dioxide from muscle to exhaled air

Introduction

This chapter deals with the anatomic system of the body in relation to the cardiac and circulatory systems (known as the cardiovascular system) from the perspective of structure, function and the effects of exercise. Instructors should be able to describe the common structures of both systems and describe their functions, as well as describe how exercise can impact on the systems.

Later chapters in the book provide physiologic and biomechanical principles that, together with the knowledge of the cardiovascular system covered in this chapter, will provide you with the understanding and ability to design appropriate exercise programs for apparently healthy individuals and to understand the effects of various types of exercise on the human body.

The cardiopulmonary system

The system that supplies oxygen and nutrients to the muscles and takes away waste products such as carbon dioxide is called the cardiopulmonary system and is made up of the lungs, the heart and associated vessels (see Figure 7.1). The lungs provide the system that deliver oxygen to and extracts carbon dioxide from the blood.

The heart

The heart is a cone-shaped organ about the size of a clenched fist and lies on the diaphragm, just left of the midline of the body. It provides a pumping service that maintains a constant circulation or blood flow to carry oxygen and carbon dioxide around the body. The wall of the heart is made up of three layers. The *myocardium* (*myo* meaning muscle), which is the middle layer, is the predominant layer and is essentially the heart muscle. The myocardium is covered on the inside by a layer of tissue known as the *endocardium* (*endo* meaning within) and on the outside by a layer of tissue known as the *epicardium* (*epi* meaning without). The entire heart is then surrounded by a fibrous tissue called the *pericardium* (*peri* meaning around), which is filled with fluid in order to protect and anchor the heart.

NEED TO KNOW

The heart beats about 100,000 times a day, or 35 million times a year, and pumps blood around an estimated 100,000 km of blood vessels.

The heart can be divided into left and right sides by a muscular wall known as the *septum*, which literally translates as 'dividing wall.' Each side contains an upper and a lower chamber. Each upper chamber is called an *atrium* (*atria* meaning entry hall) and each lower chamber is

Figure 7.1   The cardiopulmonary system

called a *ventricle* (*ventricle* meaning little belly). The left ventricle is larger and has thicker walls than the right ventricle as it pumps blood into the arteries and has to force against the pressure of the blood exerted as the arteries become progressively smaller.

Blood flow through the heart is a one-way system controlled by a number of one-way valves. The four main valves in the heart are as follows:

Atrioventricular valves

The atrioventricular valves control the flow of blood between the atrium and ventricles. The right atrioventricular valve is called the *tricuspid valve* and the left is called the *bicuspid* or *mitral valve*.

Semilunar valves

As the name suggests, semilunar valves are in the shape of a half-moon (*semi* meaning half and *lunar* meaning moon-shaped). These valves are located at the exits to arteries from the respective ventricles. The right ventricle valve, leading to the opening of the pulmonary artery, is called the *pulmonary valve* and the left ventricle valve, leading to the opening of the aorta, is called the *aortic valve*.

NEED TO KNOW

Aorte means to suspend, as it was once thought that the job of the main artery, the aorta, was to lift up the heart.

The cardiac cycle

All chambers of the heart contract and relax in a specific sequence in order to pump blood out or to fill up with blood. *Cardiac cycle* refers to this sequence of contraction and relaxation – in other words, the time taken from the start of one

NEED TO KNOW

Each heartbeat is stimulated by an elecrical impulse that originates in a small strip of heart tissue known as the sinoatrial node, or pacemaker. One of the most important advances in cardiology is the electrical pacemaker. This originates the electrical impulses when the patient's is defective.

beat to the start of another beat. The cardiac cycle can be measured by a qualified person using an ECG machine, which produces a trace known as the PQRST wave. This is essentially the trace of electrical activity across the heart during the cardiac cycle. The electrical activity in the heart is activated subconsciously by the sinoatrial node, which is a group of specialized cells in the right atrium responsible for the ordered contraction and relaxation of the heart. The sinoatrial node is also known as the natural pacemaker.

The sequence of electrical activity across the heart during a cardiac cycle is quite quick as the heart beats on average about 72 times per minute. The number of times the heart beats every minute is called the heart rate and is measured in beats per minute (bpm). The sequence of events for the cardiac cycle is as follows:

1. The 'P' section represents the contraction of the atria (atrial systole), which pumps blood into the ventricles. At this point, the ventricles are relaxed (ventricular diastole). Electrical activity is not very high as the atria do not contract strongly; this is because they are assisted by gravity and the blood is not under a large amount of pressure.
2. The 'QRS' section represents the forceful contraction of the ventricles (ventricular systole) to pump blood through the aortic and pulmonary valves into the respective vessels. This occurs about 0.1 seconds after the contraction of the atria. At this point, the valves between the atria and ventricles are closed to prevent backflow. The amount of blood pumped out of the ventricles each beat is called the *stroke volume* and the volume of blood left in the ventricles after they have contracted is called the *end systolic volume*.
3. The 'T' section is when the ventricles are relaxed and the atria are filling up prior to

their activation. The electrical activity here is returning to a resting state.

The whole cycle lasts about 0.8 seconds.

Cardiac output

The amount of blood pumped out of the heart every minute is known as the cardiac output. This can be written as follows:

Cardiac output = heart rate × stroke volume

As heart rate is measured in beats per minute (bpm) and stroke volume is measured in milliliters (ml), cardiac output is measured in milliliters per minute ($ml.min^{-1}$). Exercise can make the heart grow stronger, which could result in an increase in stroke volume as the heart can pump out more blood. As submaximal heart rate normally reduces as a long-term effect of exercise, this would mean that even though stroke volume increases, cardiac output stays relatively the same due to the reduction in heart rate.

TASK

Give a brief description of the heart and the cardiac cycle, describing any terms that you use.

Blood

Blood flow

Two *pulmonary veins* (one from each lung) carry blood that is rich in oxygen (oxygenated blood) to the left atrium in the heart. This is known as the *pulmonary circulation system.* The blood then passes through the left atrioventricular valve into the left ventricle, from where it is forcefully pumped through the aortic valve into the first (main) artery, the *aorta.*

Oxygenated blood is then pumped around a network of arteries leading to places that require it, such as muscles and organs. This is known as the *systemic circulation system.* The oxygen is passed into the muscles or organs through the smallest vessels, known as capillaries, and at the same time carbon dioxide passes from the muscles or organs into the capillaries. This exchange of gases is known as *diffusion.*

The deoxygenated blood then makes the return journey to the heart, carrying waste products such as carbon dioxide. The blood moves through a network of veins into the two main veins, called the *superior* and *inferior vena cavae.* These two veins empty the blood into the right atrium. The blood then passes through the right atrioventricular valve into the right ventricle. This process is called *venous return.*

The right ventricle then pumps the deoxygenated blood through the pulmonary valve and into the pulmonary artery. This leads back to the lungs, where carbon dioxide passes out of the capillaries into the lungs and oxygen is diffused back into the capillaries to be taken back to the left atrium via the pulmonary vein. The journey the blood makes from the right ventricle via the lungs to the left atrium is known as *pulmonary circulation.* The process then starts again. For more information on the function of the lungs, see pages 114–17.

The composition of blood

Blood is made up of straw-colored transparent fluid called *plasma* and different types of cells that are suspended in the plasma. Typically, blood contains about 55 percent plasma and 45 percent cells. The two types of cells within blood are known as red and white blood cells.

Red blood cells

Otherwise known as *erythrocytes*, red blood cells are made in the bone marrow and last for about 120 days, circulating within the body. Red blood cells contain a protein known as *hemoglobin*, which is responsible for combining with oxygen or carbon dioxide to transport it through the bloodstream. When hemoglobin combines with oxygen, it is known as *oxyhemoglobin*; when carbon dioxide is transported in the blood, it is known as *carbaminohemoglobin*.

White blood cells

Otherwise known as *leukocytes*, white blood cells are the largest of the blood cells and account for about 1 percent of the total blood volume. The main function of white blood cells is to protect the body against any foreign bodies and to remove any waste material, called *cell debris*. There are many different types of leukocytes, which have specific roles within the body.

Platelets

These are very small disks made in the red bone marrow that have a life span of between 8 and 11 days. Platelets help to prevent blood loss when a blood vessel is damaged. First, they are involved in vasoconstriction of the vessel at the damaged site and then in plugging the break. They are then involved in blood clotting at the site of the damage. When all of this occurs, the damage to the vessel can be repaired and breakdown of the clot can begin.

The circulatory system

Within the body is a network of vessels known as arteries, veins and capillaries that carry the blood and its contents to all areas. These vessels each have different functions and structures.

Arteries

With the exception of the pulmonary artery, arteries carry oxygenated blood that is under pressure away from the heart. Arteries are round with thick, elastic, muscular walls to withstand the pressure. Because of the muscular walls, arteries can get narrower (*vasoconstriction*) or open up (*vasodilation*). The space inside the artery is known as the lumen. In cases of heart disease, the lumen can become blocked by fatty deposits (*atherosclerosis*), which can then restrict blood flow and increase blood pressure. See Figure 7.2.

Arteries close to the heart are thicker than those further away due to the increased pressure they have to withstand. As the arteries branch out away from the heart, they become smaller and are known as *arterioles*. As they branch out even further, they become minute vessels called *capillaries* (see page 106).

Figure 7.2	A typical artery

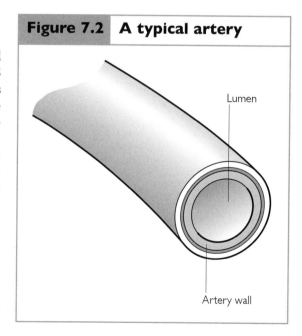

Lumen

Artery wall

Veins

With the exception of the pulmonary vein, veins carry the blood back to the heart once it has delivered oxygen to the sites that require it. In other words, veins carry deoxygenated blood. The veins are not as round as arteries and have thinner walls, as there is less pressure on them. See Figure 7.3.

Oxygenated blood flows through arteries then passes into arterioles then capillaries. The de-oxygenated blood (having given up its oxygen) then flows into vessels called venules, which in turn then flow into larger vessels called veins. As the blood that veins carry is not under as much pressure as that carried by the arteries, the veins need a system to prevent a possible backflow of blood. Veins therefore have a series of one-way valves that prevent the blood from flowing backward against the normal direction of blood flow. Other mechanisms that contribute to the overall system are gravity, muscle contraction and breathing.

Gravity

Any blood that is above the level of the heart is assisted by gravity to help it return to the heart.

Muscle contraction

Skeletal muscle contraction and smooth muscle peristaltic action help to pump blood back to the heart.

Breathing

Breathing increases pressure in the abdominal cavity, which assists blood flow back to the heart.

Capillaries

Capillaries are the smallest vessels of both arteries and veins. They are only one cell thick and porous so that carbon dioxide, oxygen and other substances can pass through in a process called *gaseous exchange*. However, red blood cells cannot pass through the capillary walls. See Figure 7.4.

Thousands of capillaries wrap around muscles so that oxygen can be delivered and carbon dioxide extracted. At the start of a network, before they branch out, capillaries have muscular sphincters (round muscles) that can open or close to either allow or prevent blood flow to the network (sometimes called *blood shunting*). These are used to ensure the areas of the body that need it the most receive oxygen at the expense of other areas. For example, when there is an increased demand for oxygen by muscles during exercise, capillary sphincters will open at the muscles doing the exercise and close in places such as the digestive system where oxygen is not required.

Figure 7.3	A typical vein

Vein wall

Figure 7.4 | A typical capillary

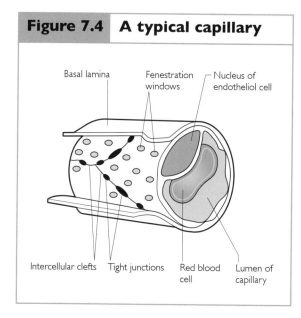

Basal lamina
Fenestration windows
Nucleus of endotheliol cell
Intercellular clefts
Tight junctions
Red blood cell
Lumen of capillary

TASK

Describe the composition of blood, the vessels that carry the blood and the method by which oxygen circulates around the body.

Blood pressure and exercise

Pressure is needed to pump the blood around the body; otherwise, it would simply gravitate to the lowest parts of the body. The pressure is greatest at the aorta as the left ventricle forcefully pumps the blood through it. By the time the blood reaches the capillaries, it is still under pressure, but not as much as in the aorta.

There are two phases of blood pressure: *systolic* and *diastolic*. Systolic pressure is the pressure on the artery walls when the ventricles contracts, and diastolic pressure is the pressure on the artery walls when the ventricles fill between beats.

The two phases of pressure can be measured to evaluate if an individual is within safe limits. The American College of Sports Medicine recommends that an average of two or more readings be taken when testing blood pressure. Table 7.1 shows the ranges for normal and high blood pressure.

If blood pressure goes above or below the normal range, it is deemed to be high or low, respectively. High blood pressure is known as *hypertension* and low blood pressure is known as *hypotension*.

Hypertension

High blood pressure can be caused by various factors, but regardless of the cause, the rate of the heart and force at which it contracts are increased to maintain the amount of blood required by the body. Long-term hypertension can result in heart attack or stroke.

Regular low-intensity aerobic exercise has been shown to reduce both systolic and

Table 7.1 | Ranges for normal and high blood pressure

	Systolic	Diastolic
Normal	120–139	80–89
High	≥140	≥90

Note: blood pressure is measured in millimeters of mercury, or mmHg diastolic blood pressure. Exercise can also prevent the tendency for blood pressure to rise. This preventive measure is important as there is less risk of heart disease in individuals who have never been hypertensive.

Hypotension

Hypotension refers to blood pressure below the normal range. Although the effects are not the same as in hypertension, individuals who have lower than normal blood pressure should be advised to move slowly when coming from a floor position to a standing position. This is because the low blood pressure can cause a reduction in blood flow to the brain due to gravity, which can cause fainting.

NEED TO KNOW

People with hypertension should avoid isometric or heavy resistance exercises as they can elevate blood pressure.

The effects of exercise on the heart

Short-term effects

Exercise leads to an increase in the rate of *cardiac output*. The stroke volume is also increased as the heart is pumping faster to supply oxygenated blood to the working muscles.

Long-term effects

The long-term effects of exercise on the heart include the following:

1. An increase in the size and strength of the cardiac muscle.
2. An increase in venous return, which reduces blood pooling.
3. Working (systolic) and resting (diastolic) blood pressure lowers, enabling the heart to work more efficiently.
4. The resting heart rate decreases.

The effects of exercise on the circulatory system

Short-term effects

The short-term effects of exercise on the circulatory system include the following:

1. Blood is diverted from non-essential areas (for example the digestive system) to the muscles that are being used.
2. Some blood vessels narrow (vasoconstrict) and some widen (vasodilate).

Long-term effects

The long-term effects of exercise on the circulatory system include the following:

1. An improvement in general circulation.
2. Vasoconstriction and vasodilation become more efficient.
3. The number of capillaries increases.
4. Greater quantities of red blood cells are produced in order to meet the requirements for an increase in the oxygen-carrying capacity of the blood.
5. There are increased levels of hemoglobin in the blood to increase the blood's capacity to bind and transport oxygen to the working muscles.

EXAMPLE QUESTIONS

7.1 The heart muscle is also known as what?

a) endocardium

b) epicardium

c) pericardium

d) myocardium

7.2 The heart muscle is covered on the inside by a layer of tissue known as what?

a) endocardium

b) epicardium

c) pericardium

d) myocardium

7.3 The entire heart muscle is covered on the outside by a layer of fibrous tissue known as what?

a) endocardium

b) epicardium

c) pericardium

d) myocardium

7.4 The mitral valve is otherwise known as the what?

a) aortic

b) tricuspid

c) bicuspid

d) semilunar

7.5 The sinoatrial node can be found in which chamber of the heart?

a) right atrium

b) left atrium

c) right ventricle

d) left ventricle

EXAMPLE QUESTIONS cont.

7.6 The aortic valve can be found in which chamber of the heart?

a) right atrium

b) left atrium

c) right ventricle

d) left ventricle

7.7 The amount of blood pumped out of the ventricles each beat is known as what?

a) end diastolic volume

b) cardiac output

c) stroke volume

d) residual volume

7.8 The amount of blood pumped out of the ventricles each beat, multiplied by the heart rate in beats per minute, is known as what?

a) end systolic volume

b) cardiac output

c) stroke volume

d) residual volume

7.9 The amount of blood left in the ventricles after each beat is known as what?

a) end diastolic volume

b) cardiac output

c) stroke volume

d) residual volume

7.10 Erythrocyte is another name for what?

a) red blood cell

b) white blood cell

c) plasma

d) platelet

EXAMPLE QUESTIONS cont.

7.11 Leukocyte is another name for what?
a) red blood cell
b) white blood cell
c) plasma
d) platelet

7.12 Which of the following makes up the largest percentage of volume in the blood?
a) red blood cells
b) white blood cells
c) plasma
d) platelets

Further reading

Abrahams, P., Craven, J. and Lumley, J. (2005) *Illustrated Clinical Anatomy*, Hodder Arnold

American College of Sports Medicine (2006) *Guidelines to Exercise Testing and Prescription* (7th ed.), Lippincott, Williams & Wilkins

Baechle, R.T. (2000) *Essentials of Strength Training and Conditioning* (2nd ed.), Human Kinetics

Marieb, E.N. (2001) *Human Anatomy and Physiology*, Benjamin Cummings

Porter, S. (2002) *The Anatomy Workbook*, Butterworth Heinemann

Sewell, D., Watkins, P. and Griffin, M. (2005) *Sport and Exercise Science: An Introduction*, Hodder Arnold

Tortora, G.J. and Grabowski, S.R. (2003) *Principles of Anatomy and Physiology* (10th ed.), Wiley

Wilson, K.J.W. and Waugh, A. (1998) *Ross and Wilson Anatomy and Physiology in Health and Illness*, Churchill Livingstone

NOTES

THE RESPIRATORY SYSTEM

8

OBJECTIVES

After completing this chapter, you will be able to

1 Describe the structure of the lungs in relation to their function.

2 Explain the passage of air into and out of the lungs.

3 Explain the process of exchange of gases.

4 List the percentages of gases in inspired and expired air.

5 Explain the mechanism of breathing.

Instructing Exercise and Fitness Knowledge

Basic Anatomy and Physiology

■ The location and function of the lungs and capillaries.

■ The short- and long-term effects of exercise on the respiratory system.

Instructing Physical Activity and Exercise Knowledge

Anatomy: The Respiratory System

■ Anatomy of the lungs:

  • Structure of the lungs and airways
  • Inspiration and expiration (including the role of the diaphragm and intercostal muscles)
  • Breathing regulation (respiratory center – hypothalamus)
  • Effect of smoking on the lungs

■ Pathway of oxygen from inhaled air to muscle

■ Pathway of carbon dioxide from muscle to exhaled air

Introduction

This chapter deals with the anatomic system of the body in relation to the respiratory system from the perspective of structure, function and the effects of exercise. Instructors should be able to describe the common structures of the respiratory system and describe the function of the system, as well as describe how exercise can impact on the system.

Later chapters in the book provide physiologic and biomechanical principles that, together with the knowledge of the cardiovascular system covered in the previous chapter and the respiratory system covered in this chapter, provide you with the understanding and ability to design appropriate exercise programs for apparently healthy individuals and to understand the effects of various types of exercise on the human body.

The respiratory system

The *respiratory system* is the collective term given to the nose, pharynx, larynx, trachea, bronchi and lungs. Essentially, it filters, warms and moistens air before conducting it to the lungs, which house specific sites where gases are exchanged between the air and the blood. See Figure 8.1.

The lungs

The lungs are a pair of cone-shaped organs made of elastic tissue that expand to allow air from the atmosphere to enter. They are roughly level with the heart in the thoracic cavity and are surrounded by a double membrane called the *pleura*. Each lung has a superior (upper), middle and inferior (lower) lobe.

Figure 8.1   The respiratory system

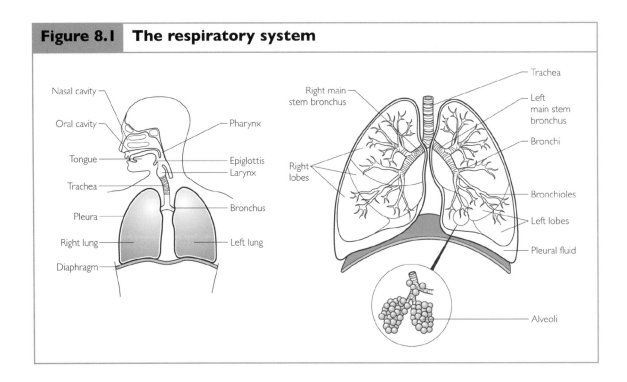

The passage of air

Air that is breathed in is known as *inspired air*, whereas air that is breathed out is called *expired air*. Air is made up of various gases, and the composition of gases in inspired air is different from that of expired air (see Table 8.1). About 5 percent of the oxygen in inspired air is used up, so expired air contains less oxygen. About 4 percent carbon dioxide is produced during breathing, so expired air has more carbon dioxide than inspired air.

The *passage of air* describes how oxygen from the air reaches the muscles that require it for the production of energy. First, air is taken in through the mouth or the nose. If the air is passed through the nose, it can be warmed, moistened and filtered; this occurs to a lesser extent to air taken in through the mouth, which can induce asthmatic reactions. The air then passes through the *pharynx* (throat), which lies behind the nose and the mouth and is a passage for food and air. The pharynx is lined with a mucous membrane that provides moisture, and the wall of the pharynx is made of skeletal muscle (see pages 38–41). The pharynx also houses the tonsils, which play a part in reactions against foreign invaders such as viruses.

The air then passes down through the *larynx* (voice box), which extends to the level of the start of the thoracic vertebrae. The air is continually warmed and moistened as it travels through the larynx. The larynx wall is made up of several pieces of cartilage connected by muscle tissue. One of the pieces of cartilage is known as the *epiglottis* (*epi* meaning over and *glottis* meaning tongue), which is essentially a trapdoor that controls the passage of air and food (it closes when swallowing to prevent food and drink going into the airways). From the larynx, the air continues into a rigid cartilaginous tube called the *trachea* (*trachea* meaning sturdy) or windpipe, which is lined with fine hairs that filter the air. The trachea runs down to the level of the fifth thoracic vertebra, where it divides into the left and right *bronchi*.

NEED TO KNOW

The thyroid cartilage is a small piece of cartilage at the front of the throat, otherwise known as the Adam's apple. Its role is to influence the tension of the vocal cords and is usually larger in males, which is why men have deeper voices than women.

Air passes into each of the bronchi, which enter the left and right lungs and split into smaller bronchi. These then split into smaller tubes called *bronchioles*, which in turn branch out and finally lead into air sacs called *alveoli*. The alveoli then fill up with air and expand to a size dependent on

Table 8.1	Composition of inspired and expired air	
	Inspired air (%)	Expired air (%)
Oxygen	21	16
Carbon dioxide	0.04	4
Nitrogen	78	78

breathing levels and other physical factors. It is here that gaseous exchange takes place so that oxygen can enter the bloodstream to be transported to working muscles and carbon dioxide can be removed from the bloodstream in expired air. The amount of air remaining in the lungs after a maximal breath out is known as the *residual volume*.

NEED TO KNOW

Sometimes the airflow through the trachea can become blocked. Therefore, an incision is made through the wall of the trachea and a tube is inserted so that the patient can breathe. This is known as a tracheostomy.

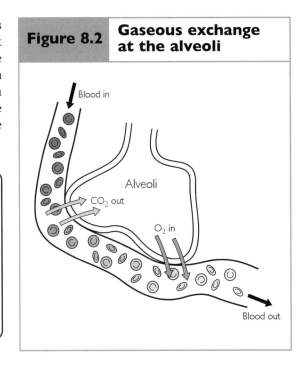

Figure 8.2 **Gaseous exchange at the alveoli**

Gaseous exchange

In order for oxygen to pass from the alveoli into the bloodstream, it must first pass through the walls of the alveoli. All alveoli are surrounded by numerous capillaries, which then lead into the network of veins and arteries. Oxygen can pass through the membrane wall of the alveoli and through the wall of the capillaries as both structures are only one cell thick. Carbon dioxide passes the opposite way, from the capillaries into the alveoli, to be breathed out (see Figure 8.2).

This exchange of gases is possible due to the *pressure gradient*. In general terms, gases pass from an area of high concentration (or pressure) to an area of low concentration in order to equalize the concentration. For example, after breathing in (*inspiration*) there is a higher concentration of oxygen in the alveoli than in the capillaries surrounding them, so the oxygen diffuses from the alveoli to the capillaries. Likewise, there is a higher concentration of

carbon dioxide in the capillaries than in the alveoli, so the carbon dioxide diffuses from the capillaries into the alveoli.

Breathing control

One of the main factors involved in breathing control is the level of carbon dioxide in the blood. When the amount of carbon dioxide in the blood reaches a certain level, respiratory centers in the brain stem activate breathing muscles via the central nervous system.

Generally, the breathing rate (the number of breaths per minute) is about 12 times per minute. This increases during exercise as the demand for more oxygen by the working muscles is recognized by the respiratory center in the brain stem, which in turn increases the number of breaths per minute. Therefore, in this way the breathing rate is controlled subconsciously. Breathing can also be controlled consciously.

The amount of air taken into the lungs during a normal breath is called the *tidal volume*. The maximum amount of air breathed out after a maximal inspiration is called the *vital capacity* and is sometimes measured to monitor progress during an exercise program although it is mainly used to identify possible lung disease.

The role of muscles in breathing

The main muscles involved in breathing in (inspiration) when an individual is not involved in exercise are the diaphragm and the external intercostals. The scalenes and the pectoralis minor contribute during vigorous exercise.

Expiration (breathing out) is predominantly passive as the result of *elastic recoil* by certain tissues: tissues such as muscles have a certain amount of elasticity, which means they will return to their prestretched state when the contraction stops. The muscles involved in expiration are the internal intercostals and certain abdominal muscles. During forced expiration (breathing heavily), the transversus abdominis is also used.

NEED TO KNOW

When your stomach aches after laughing forcefully it is usually due to fatigue of the transversus abdominis, which is not used to working so hard.

TASK

List and describe the structures of the respiratory system and explain how oxygen and carbon dioxide are exchanged between the air and the blood.

The effects of smoking on the respiratory system

The exact mechanisms of the effects of smoking on the respiratory system are complicated and are still being investigated in current research. However, a summary of the effects is given below:

1. Tar from cigarettes can remain in the alveoli, which can restrict the amount of air taken in.
2. Cigarette smoke can destroy the alveoli wall, which prevents the diffusion of oxygen and carbon dioxide.
3. Smoking is one of the leading causes of chronic bronchitis, which is the inflammation of the airways leading to a restriction in the passage of air.
4. Smoking is one of the most common causes of lung cancer. Most people with lung cancer die within the first year of diagnosis.
5. Pneumonia, which relates to inflammation of the alveoli, can be caused by smoking.
6. Nicotine from cigarettes narrows the smaller airways, which can decrease the airflow.
7. Hemoglobin (the oxygen carrier in the blood) prefers to carry carbon monoxide from smoke rather than oxygen, which reduces its oxygen-carrying capacity.
8. Smoking can cause increased mucus secretion and destroy the lining of the airways.

The effects of exercise on the respiratory system

Short-term effects

The short-term effects of exercise on the respiratory system include the following:

1. The rate of exchange of gases within the lungs increases, as does the volume of gases exchanged.

2. Levels of carbon dioxide in the body increase, so more has to be removed.
3. The depth of breathing increases, followed by the rate of breathing.

Long-term effects

The long-term effects of exercise on the respiratory system include the following:

1. The respiratory muscles become stronger.
2. Gaseous exchange at the alveoli takes place more easily.
3. The breathing effort required decreases.
4. The number of capillaries increases.

EXAMPLE QUESTIONS

8.1 Air sacs in the lungs are also known as what?
a) alveoli
b) pleura
c) bronchioles
d) capillaries

8.2 The double membrane surrounding the lungs is known as what?
a) alveoli
b) pleura
c) bronchioles
d) capillaries

8.3 Gaseous exchange takes place between what?
a) alveoli and capillaries
b) pleura and capillaries
c) bronchioles and alveoli
d) pleura and alveoli

8.4 What is the percentage difference of oxygen between inspired and expired air?
a) 17
b) 21
c) 5
d) 78

8.5 The amount of air left in the lungs after a maximal expiration is known as what?
a) expiratory ratio
b) tidal volume
c) residual volume
d) vital capacity

EXAMPLE QUESTIONS cont.

8.6 The maximum amount of air breathed out of the lungs after a maximum breath in is known as what?

a) expiratory ratio

b) tidal volume

c) residual volume

d) vital capacity

8.7 Which of the following gases can stimulate breathing when blood levels reach a certain point?

a) helium

b) carbon dioxide

c) nitrogen

d) hydrogen

8.8 The amount of air taken into the lungs during a normal breath is called what?

a) expiratory ratio

b) tidal volume

c) residual volume

d) vital capacity

8.9 The voice box is otherwise known as what?

a) larynx

b) pharynx

c) trachea

d) bronchiole

8.10 The windpipe is otherwise known as what?

a) larynx

b) pharynx

c) trachea

d) bronchiole

EXAMPLE QUESTIONS cont.

8.11 Which of the following lead directly into the alveoli?

a) larynx

b) pharynx

c) trachea

d) bronchiole

8.12 Which of the following structures is only one cell thick?

a) pleural membrane

b) trachea

c) bronchioles

d) capillaries

Further reading

Abrahams, P., Craven, J. and Lumley, J. (2005) *Illustrated Clinical Anatomy*, Hodder Arnold

Baechle, R.T. (2000) *Essentials of Strength Training and Conditioning* (2nd ed.), Human Kinetics

Marieb, E.N. (2001) *Human Anatomy and Physiology*, Benjamin Cummings

Porter, S. (2002) *The Anatomy Workbook*, Butterworth Heinemann

Sewell, D., Watkins, P. and Griffin, M. (2005) *Sport and Exercise Science: An Introduction*, Hodder Arnold

Tortora, G.J. and Grabowski, S.R. (2003) *Principles of Anatomy and Physiology* (10th ed.), Wiley

Wilson, K.J.W. and Waugh, A. (1998) *Ross and Wilson Anatomy and Physiology in Health and Illness*, Churchill Livingstone

NOTES

CORE STABILITY

OBJECTIVES

After completing this chapter, you will be able to

1   Define the terms 'stabilizer' and 'mobilizer' in relation to muscle roles.

2   Identify muscles known as local and global.

3   List the methods of spinal stabilization.

4   Define 'neutral zone' and explain the teaching methods related to this.

5   Explain the principle of intra-abdominal pressure.

6   Describe the process for the contraction of the transversus abdominis.

7   List and describe common stability exercises.

Instructing Exercise and Fitness Knowledge

Basic Anatomy and Physiology

- The structure and range of movement of the spine.

- The types of muscular contraction; location and action of major muscle groups; how voluntary muscles contract.

- The effect of speed on posture, alignment and intensity.

- The needs and potential of the participant, including reasons for and barriers to participation in the appropriate activity.

- Exercises that are safe and appropriate for participants, including alternatives to potentially harmful exercises; safe and effective alignment of exercise positions.

- Reasons for temporary deferral of exercise; referral; informed consent.

Instructing Physical Activity and Exercise Knowledge

Anatomy: Functional Kinesiology

- Postural muscles and core stability

- Anatomy of muscular and mechanical systems associated with core stability:

- Local and global stabilizing muscles
- Fiber type overview of local and global muscles
- Fundamental principles of core stabilization:
  - Rationale for stabilization to exist because of excessive forces on the spine
  - Neutral zone control from the muscular system
  - Intra-abdominal pressure and its role in stabilization
  - Thoracolumbar fascia and its role in stabilization
  - Abdominal bracing and its role in stabilization
  - The glute complex and its role in stabilization of the spine and reducing the risk of low back pain
  - The use of stabilization equipment
- Exercises associated with core stabilization:
  - Methods of contraction of the transversus abdominis
  - Methods of abdominal bracing
  - Stability equipment exercises
  - Floor-based exercises
  - Reasons for participant exclusion

Introduction

This chapter deals with the anatomic system of the body, in particular the structure and function of muscles associated with spinal stability. The chapter also deals with commonly prescribed exercises for short- and long-term development of the associated muscles. Instructors should be able to identify the muscular system associated with spinal, or core, stabilization and describe their functions, as well as describe how exercise can impact on efficiency and development.

Other chapters in the book provide some of the physiologic and biomechanical principles that, together with the specific theory covered in this chapter, will provide you with the understanding and ability to design appropriate exercise programs for apparently healthy individuals and to understand the effects of various types of exercise on the human body.

Core stability

In simple terms, core stability is the process of holding the shoulder and pelvic girdles (that is the center part, or core of the body) stable in order to support the movement forces from the arms and legs. In order to do this, the muscles that are responsible for the stabilizing role must function correctly in order that the muscles responsible for movement are able to perform their function correctly. Unfortunately, in many people the muscles responsible for stabilizing and movement have become less than efficient due to a number of factors associated with poor posture. Everyday tasks such as sitting in cars, at desks and on sofas have led to the stabilizing muscles becoming weaker, as the objects we sit on take on the role of stabilizing and support. As a result, other muscles that are usually associated with movement tasks take on the role of stabilization. This can lead to weakness in certain movements and can eventually cause muscle, tendon or ligament injury, especially in cases where the speed of a movement is increased. In turn, this will increase the possibility of injury due to the greater demand for stabilization.

NEED TO KNOW

Everybody is capable of a certain degree of core stabilization. However, in most cases specific muscles need to be retrained to perform the role that they are physiologically best suited for.

Stabilizers and mobilizers

The everyday demands placed on the posture and control of the human body mean that the muscles responsible for core stabilization (*stabilizers*; also known as *tonic muscles*) are designed to perform endurance tasks rather than short-term or explosive tasks. These muscles are sometimes described as 'nature's corset' and are required to carry out a stabilizing role for long periods of time. Due to the demands of these endurance-type tasks, stabilizers are predominantly made up of type I slow-twitch fibers (see page 44).

In a normal functional person, while the role of stabilization is being undertaken muscles known as *mobilizers* are able to carry out their role of locomotion or movement of the body. These muscles are usually required to provide a short-term or *phasic* role and are therefore not classed as endurance muscles. Mobilizer muscles are often found to be predominantly made up of fast-twitch fibers and are more superficial (closer to the surface) than stabilizer muscles.

It is commonplace for stabilizing and mobilizing muscles to be trained to perform the opposite role from that which they were designed for. For example, the rectus abdominis is predominantly a fast-twitch muscle close to the surface of the body and is normally active in strength or explosive tasks, such as running and jumping where the legs come toward the torso (spinal flexion). However, it is common for exercise programs to include sit-up type exercises that are performed repetitively in an endurance-type capacity. The rectus abdominis is mainly responsible for this sit-up action, which effectively results in a predominantly fast-twitch muscle taking on the role of a slow-twitch muscle. This often weakens the stabilizer muscles as the rectus abdominis has taken on this role. The drawback of this is that the rectus abdominis tries to perform both stabilizing and mobilizing roles, potentially leading to back pain or injury as optimal stabilization of the spine is not performed. This reversal of roles is a common problem in exercise programs for many different muscles within the body.

Inner and outer units

Current research seems to suggest that both deep and superficial muscles in the trunk and pelvic region contribute in some way to spinal stabilization (Richardson et al., 2003). What is not clear is the extent to which the general population has limited function of one or both of the systems.

Muscles in the body that are deep are sometimes referred to as *local muscles* or, in relation to core stabilization, as the *inner unit*. The transversus abdominis, multifidus, pelvic floor, diaphragm and internal obliques are all examples of local muscles. Muscles that are superficial are commonly known as *global muscles* or the *outer unit*. The rectus abdominis, external obliques and some parts of the erector spinae are all global muscles. At the hip joint, the gluteus maximus and gluteus minimus are usually considered to be mobilizers and the gluteus medius is normally considered to be a stabilizer. There are many other muscles associated with stabilization of the hip complex, but the main ones are mentioned above. The main muscles of the inner unit are listed below.

Transversus abdominis

This muscle forms a belt or corset around the trunk region and lies deep below the rectus abdominis muscle, which is associated with the 'six-pack.' Imagine a belt running underneath the navel, right around the body. This is the transversus abdominis muscle. See Figure 9.1.

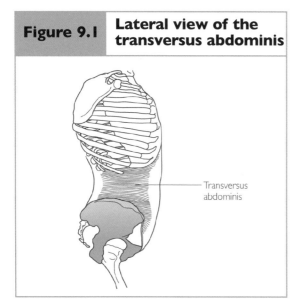

Figure 9.1 | **Lateral view of the transversus abdominis**

Transversus abdominis

Multifidus

This is a series of many small muscles that attach between each vertebra of the spine (see Figure 9.2). These muscles act as a kind of lashing for the bones in the spine to prevent any excessive movement.

Figure 9.2 | **Posterior view of the multifidus**

Multifidus

Internal obliques

These attach from the lower ribs and insert into the pubic bone, and lie at an angle just above and below the navel (see Figure 9.3). They are quite deep and cannot be seen superficially.

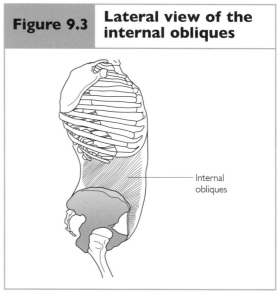

Figure 9.3 | **Lateral view of the internal obliques**

Internal obliques

Pelvic floor

The pelvic floor muscles run from the coccyx (bones at the bottom of the spine), under the crotch area to the pubic bone at the front (see Figure 9.4).

Diaphragm

This is a dome-shaped muscle that covers the region under the ribcage (see Figure 9.5). As well as performing core stabilization tasks, the diaphragm is responsible for helping in breathing movements.

The inner unit or local muscles are predominantly slow-twitch (tonic) and are responsible for stabilizing the core of the body, in particular the spine. The outer unit or global muscles are predominantly fast-twitch (phasic) and are mainly responsible for movement, although they do contribute in a limited way to stabilization.

In order for the spine to remain protected at all times, it is essential that both the inner and

| Figure 9.5 | **Anterior view of the diaphragm** |

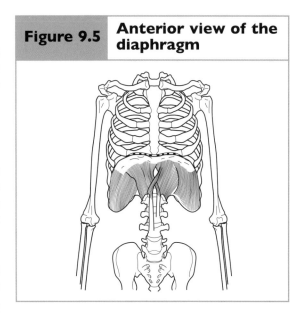

outer units are working optimally. The ability of both units to function correctly is somewhat dependent on information relayed by the neuromuscular system. If this is not functioning optimally, the inner and outer units will not function optimally. Table 9.1 provides an overview of common local and global muscles and their characteristics.

TASK

Give a brief definition of the term 'core stabilization' and describe the differences between stabilizing and mobilizing muscles in relation to inner and outer units.

Mechanisms of stabilization

It has been demonstrated that, even when lifting small loads, the spine as a column would collapse if it did not have any form of support

| Figure 9.4 | **The pelvic floor muscles** |

Bowel

Womb

Bladder

Pubic bone

Pelvic floor muscles

Table 9.1	Common characteristics of local and global muscles	
	Local muscles (transversus abdominis, multifidus, pelvic floor, diaphragm, internal obliques)	Global muscles (rectus abdominis, external obliques, erector spinae)
Main fiber type	Slow-twitch	Fast-twitch
General task	Postural/endurance	Strength/explosive
Location	Deep	Superficial
Role	Stabilizing	Mobilizing
Common contraction	Isometric	Eccentric and concentric

or stabilization. The mechanisms of stabilization of the spine (core stability) are not fully understood, but it is thought that several systems, in conjunction with the ligaments of the spine, contribute to its overall stabilization. Systems such as *intra-abdominal pressure, thoracolumbar fascia gain* and the *hydraulic amplifier effect* are thought to provide enough spinal stabilization for the body to carry out normal daily tasks. However, although the spine and its stabilization systems are capable of protecting the spine under normal circumstances, an overload due to certain exercises, sport or poor posture can lead to a dysfunction in one or more of the systems, which could in turn lead to injury.

Intra-abdominal pressure

In order to achieve an effective degree of core stability, the stabilizing muscles of the inner unit must activate and contract together to help make the trunk more solid. This can be achieved in a number of ways, one of which is a process called intra-abdominal pressure.

The contents of the trunk area, including the stomach, intestines and various organs and fluid, are collectively termed the *abdominal ball* or *fluid ball*, which is cylinder-like in shape. When the core muscles contract, the walls of the abdominal ball are tightened and compressed, which creates an increase in pressure known as intra-abdominal pressure. This pushes against the spine and prevents it from making any excessive movements, and helps to keep the spine in the correct posture (see Figure 9.6).

The example of an airbag inflated in a driver's seat can help to explain the process. It is difficult for the driver to move against the airbag as the pressure resists his or her movement. The same principle applies with intra-abdominal pressure, where the abdominal ball resists the movements of the spine. In effect, this encourages the spine to move as a complete unit and prevents one part of the spine moving across another part of the spine, which could easily lead to injury.

The main muscles responsible for intra-abdominal pressure are the transversus abdominis, the internal obliques and the multifidus muscles, which form the walls of the abdominal ball; the diaphragm, which forms the top of the abdominal ball; and the pelvic floor muscle, which forms the base of the abdominal ball. It is important that all of these muscles contract together so that the increase in pressure is evenly distributed along the spine. This requires an element of control, which is sometimes lost through lack of practice. It therefore requires a conscious effort and a lot of practice to achieve this contraction of the inner unit.

NEED TO KNOW

Researchers have found that in people with chronic low back pain the inner unit muscles do not function correctly. Dysfunction of the inner unit could be one of the causes of low back pain.

Thoracolumbar fascia gain

The *thoracolumbar fascia* is a sheet of connective tissue, almost tendon-like, that covers most of the muscles in the back and attaches to the spine, pelvis and sacrum. When the muscles of the inner unit are activated, tension is produced in the thoracolumbar fascia. It has been suggested that this tension creates an extension force on the spine (in other words, causes it to stiffen) and thus provides a degree of stabilization that contributes to the overall stabilization of the spine. The exact mechanism of thoracolumbar fascia gain is still under investigation and a topic of much debate.

Hydraulic amplifier effect

When the erector spinae muscles contract, the thoracolumbar fascia that surrounds these muscles resists their expansion. This resistance increases the strength of the erector spinae muscles by up to 30 percent, and therefore it can be assumed that this effect contributes in some way to the stabilization of the spine. Again, like thoracolumbar fascia gain, the hydraulic amplifier effect is currently being researched and the exact mechanisms are not yet fully understood.

TASK

Briefly explain the mechanisms that contribute to the overall stabilization of the spine.

Neutral position or zone

The concept of the neutral position of the spine can be explained by thinking about the gears in a car. When a car is in neutral, there is no torque, or turning force on the transmission. However, when the gears are engaged, considerable force is applied to make the car move. Similarly, when a normal functional spine is in its *neutral zone* (also known as *neutral spine*), which is approximately midway between full posterior and anterior tilts of the pelvis (see pages 131–32), minimal force is placed on the spine and the structures that surround it (tendons, cartilage and ligaments). Any movement away from this position dramatically increases the stress placed on the surrounding tissues and hence the spine itself. Stabilization control to maintain neutral spine is required when carrying out simple tasks such as sitting, as well as performing more complex tasks such as changing direction while running at speed, in order to prevent undue stress on the surrounding tissues that might eventually lead to injury. As mentioned above, this stabilization control appears to be lacking in the majority of people who suffer from back pain and is thought to be one of the major causes of the back pain or injury responsible for the pain.

Awareness of the body and the position of its segments is a complex skill that requires practice – something that is made evident by the number of people who display poor posture. What appears to be neutral spine to an individual may not be considered neutral by the observer. Neutral spine can be found with the help of an observer by either standing or sitting on a stability ball and tilting the pelvis back and forward until the neutral position is found (see below). Tilting the pelvis forward (anterior tilt) increases the hollow in the lumbar spine area, whereas tilting the pelvis backward (posterior tilt) flattens the lumbar spine area. This method of finding neutral spine is not an exact science but can be used to help the general population gain an awareness of posture.

Seated procedure for finding the neutral zone

Practitioner

1. Sit in an upright position on the stability ball with the knee joint just below the level of the hip joint and the feet shoulder-width apart.
2. Attempt to flatten the lower spine by pulling the crotch area up toward the chest (posterior tilt – see Figure 9.6a).
3. Attempt to increase the hollow in the lower back by pulling the buttocks in a straight line toward the shoulder blades (posterior tilt – see Figure 9.6b).
4. Repeat this movement several times at a slow, controlled pace.
5. Try to find the neutral position, after being informed of the correct position by the observer (see Figure 9.6c).

Observer

1. Make sure that any movement occurs only in the lumbar spine; do not allow any movement at the shoulders or in the legs.
2. Watch for the full range of motion between the full anterior and the full posterior tilt.

Inform the practitioner when the pelvis is midway between these two points.

Figure 9.6 **(a–c) Seated procedure for finding the neutral spine**

(a)

(b)

(c)

Standing procedure for finding the neutral zone

Practitioner

1. Stand in an upright position with the feet shoulder-width apart.
2. Attempt to flatten the lower spine by pulling the crotch area up towards the chest. (See Figure 9.7a.)
3. Attempt to increase the hollow in the lower back by pulling the buttocks in a straight line towards the shoulder blades. (See Figure 9.7b.)
4. Repeat this movement several times at a slow, controlled pace.
5. Try to find the neutral position after being informed of the correct position by the observer. (See Figure 9.7c.)

Observer

1. Make sure that any movement occurs only in the lumbar spine; do not allow any movement at the shoulders or in the legs.
2. Watch for the full range of motion between the full anterior and the full posterior tilt.
3. Inform the practitioner when the pelvis is midway between these two points.

NEED TO KNOW

To help prevent any unwanted movement, the observer can place both hands on the shoulders of the practitioner. The observer will feel any unwanted movement.

| Figure 9.7 | **(a–c) Standing procedure for finding the neutral spine** |

(a)

(b)

(c)

Contraction of the transversus abdominis

One of the mechanisms that can be used to achieve stabilization of the spine is the principle known as the 'abdominal' or 'fluid ball' technique. Through the contraction of certain stabilizing muscles, pressure is placed upon the spine, which prevents unwanted movement and helps the spine to work as a unit. It would be almost impossible to consciously contract all of the muscles associated with stabilization. When the transversus abdominis muscle is contracted either consciously or subconsciously, the other muscles of the inner unit contract immediately afterward.

Contraction of the stabilizing muscles (inner unit) can be very difficult for several reasons. Many years of misuse, poor posture, overuse and weakness can result in a lack of subconscious activation of these muscles. As a result, it is common for exercises to be taught that are designed to improve subconscious activation of the inner unit muscles. One of the main difficulties associated with conscious activation is that many individuals try too hard, which usually results in the holding of breath and an increase in blood pressure. Research has suggested that only 30 percent of the maximum contraction capability of the inner unit muscles is needed to create sufficient intra-abdominal pressure to stabilize the spine (Richardson et al., 2003).

Contraction of the transversus abdominis can be one of the most difficult conscious tasks for an individual to perform. However, for the contraction of the stabilizing muscles to become subconscious (autonomous), it is essential to perform conscious practice of muscle contraction on a regular basis. The following method may be used to practice contraction of the transversus muscle, which will in turn activate the other stabilizing muscles.

Conscious activation of the transversus abdominis

Body position

Lie with your back on the floor, knees bent and feet flat on the floor. Relax and try not to flatten the spine against the floor; instead, maintain a normal lumbar curve.

Hand position

Find a position 2 inches below the navel and 2 inches to either side of that position. Press in lightly on each side using the first two fingers of each hand. This should be the location of the transversus abdominis. Slide one hand under the natural curve of the lower spine so that you can feel any pressure changes from the body through the hand.

Initial contraction

Cough! As the transversus abdominis is one of the muscles responsible for the forced expiration of air during coughing, you should feel the contraction under your fingers, that is you should feel the muscle getting harder. The pressure on the hand under the lumbar spine should not change. Try to maintain constant pressure throughout the contraction.

Practice

The aim of the exercise is to try to replicate the contraction felt when coughing, without actually coughing. This can sometimes take a considerable amount of time to achieve, but once you can do it aim to contract at about 30 percent of your maximum contraction capability.

Progression

Once you can contract the transversus abdominis, perform the same action without holding your breath or activating the rectus abdominis (a common mistake found in most people). You can place a hand just below the diaphragm to check for contraction of the rectus abdominis.

The lying method of contraction is suitable for initial purposes. Once individuals are capable of contracting their transversus abdominis, use the same method in a standing position. This makes it easier for individuals to perform the exercise on a daily basis.

The length of time, number of repetitions and frequency of practice of conscious contraction required to develop subconscious contraction control are different for every individual. It can be a lengthy process lasting up to several months, so it is recommended that conscious contraction practice be maintained for a period of no less than six months.

Typical core stability exercises

Once individuals are capable of contracting the transversus abdominis by conscious control, they can progress to other types of common stabilization exercises. Individuals with no history of performing stabilization exercises should initially be prescribed the most basic exercises and should only progress to more difficult exercises when they are comfortable with the previous level of stabilization exercise.

The following core stability exercises should not be prescribed to clients who have back problems or who report pain when performing the exercises. Simple screening procedures (see Chapter 11) should be sufficient to identify individuals who should not be prescribed stabilization exercises. The exercises might need to be deferred until the individual has been referred to a doctor and has been authorized to carry out an exercise program.

Floor exercises

Kneeling abdominal hollow

See Figure 9.8.

Starting position

1. Kneel on the floor with your shoulders directly above your hands and your hips directly above your knees.
2. Keep your head facing down toward the floor to prevent undue stress on the cervical spine.
3. Keep your knees shoulder-width apart. Check that your spine is in the neutral position.

Action

1. Consciously contract your transversus abdominis.
2. Breathe gently in and out, maintaining the contraction.

3. Breathe out and, before breathing in again, try to hollow your lower abdominals (imagine pulling your navel toward your spine).
4. Continuing to breathe normally, hold this position for a few seconds or until you are unable to hold it any more.
5. Repeat, trying to maintain normal breathing throughout.
6. Concentrate on maintaining the starting position during the course of the exercise.

Progressions

1. Try to perform the action without contracting the rectus abdominis.
2. Once you are comfortable with performing abdominal hollowing on all fours, try to perform the action in a standing position.
3. Try to contract the transversus abdominis without drawing in the lower abdominals. This is known as *abdominal bracing*.

Figure 9.8 | **Kneeling abdominal hollow**

Supine foot slide

See Figures 9.9a and b.

Starting position

1. Lie on your back with your feet flat on the floor and your knees bent as much as is comfortably possible.
2. Place one arm down by your side and the other under the lumbar spine to check the pressure on your hand throughout the exercise.
3. Keep your knees shoulder-width apart. Check that your spine is in the neutral position.

Action

1. Consciously contract your transversus abdominis.

2. Breathe gently in and out.
3. Slowly slide one foot outward along the floor until your leg is fully extended.
4. Return to the start position, trying to maintain normal breathing throughout.
5. Concentrate on keeping your spine in the neutral position during the exercise so that the pressure on your hand does not change.

Progressions

1. Once you are comfortable with the above action, try increasing the speed of the movement slightly.
2. Once you can perform the above exercise without a change in pressure on the hand under the lumbar spine, try sliding both legs out and back at the same time.

Figure 9.9 **(a) and (b) Supine foot slide**

(a)

(b)

Pelvic tilts

See Figures 9.10a and b.

Starting position

1. Lie on your back with your feet flat on the floor and your knees bent as much as is comfortably possible.
2. Place your arms by your sides or across your abdomen.
3. Keep your knees shoulder-width apart. Check that your spine is in the neutral position.

Action

1. Consciously contract your transversus abdominis.
2. Breathe in and out gently.
3. Tilt your pelvis backward so that your lower back is flat on the floor (see Figure 9.10b).
4. Return to the starting position, trying to maintain normal breathing throughout.

Progressions

1. Try performing the exercise while lifting one foot slightly off the floor.
2. As well as tilting the pelvis backward, try to tilt it forward so that your lumbar spine is more arched than normal.

Figure 9.10 | **(a) and (b) Pelvic tilts**

(a) (b)

Side bridge

See Figures 9.11a and b.

Starting position

1. Lie on your side with your feet slightly apart to create a stable base.
2. Bend the arm nearest the floor at the elbow and rest it on the floor. This will provide support when you lift your upper body off the floor.
3. Put the opposite arm down by your side. Check that your spine is in the neutral position.
4. Keep your upper hip in line with your lower hip (see Figure 9.11a).

Action

1. Consciously contract your transversus abdominis.

2. Breathe gently in and out.
3. Raise your lower hip off the floor so that your body forms a straight line (see Figure 9.11b).
4. Hold this position until you start to feel muscle fatigue.
5. Try to maintain normal breathing throughout.
6. Concentrate on keeping your spine in the neutral position during the exercise.

Progression

Once you are comfortable with the above exercise, start with the hip in the raised position. Try to lower the hip nearest the floor toward the floor and then raise it to the start position again. Repeat.

Figure 9.11 (a) and (b) Side bridge

(a)

(b)

Stability ball exercises

Shoulder bridge

See Figure 9.12.

Starting position

1. Sit upright on the ball.
2. Walk your feet forward and lean back at the same time until the ball is under your shoulder blades.
3. Lie face up with the ball under your shoulder blades.
4. Rest your head back onto the ball.
5. Keep your feet shoulder-width apart and your arms outstretched with the palms facing down.
6. Check that your spine is in the neutral position.
7. Keep a straight horizontal line through your shoulder, knee and hip joints.

Action

1. Consciously contract your transversus abdominis.
2. With your feet shoulder-width apart and your arms outstretched, gently roll a few inches to one side at the shoulders and then return to the starting point.
3. Repeat, but roll to the opposite side.
4. Repeat this five times to each side.
5. Maintain normal breathing throughout.
6. Concentrate on maintaining the starting position during the exercise.

Safety point

Roll only as far as you feel in control of the movement. Use your hands to prevent yourself rolling if you go too far.

Figure 9.12	Shoulder bridge

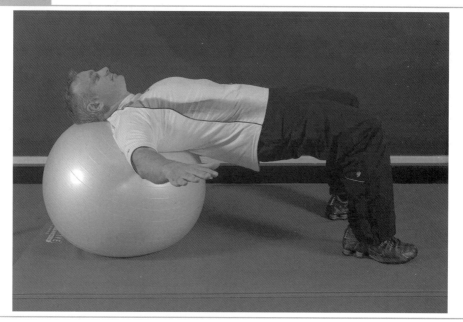

Foot bridge

See Figure 9.13.

Starting position

1. Lie face up on the floor.
2. Place the soles of your feet midway between the top and the side of the ball.
3. Keep your feet shoulder-width apart and your arms outstretched.
4. Raise your bottom off the floor until your spine is in the neutral position. Your knee joints should be at about 90 degrees at this point.
5. Only your shoulder blades, head and arms should be resting on the floor.

Action

1. Consciously contract your transversus abdominis.
2. With your feet shoulder-width apart and your arms outstretched, use your feet to roll the ball gently a few inches to one side and then return to the starting point.
3 Repeat, but roll to the opposite side.
4. Repeat five times to each side.
5. Maintain normal breathing throughout.
6. Concentrate on maintaining the starting position during the exercise.

Safety point

Roll only as far as you feel in control of the movement. If you lose control, adopt the starting position and repeat from the point at which you lost control.

Figure 9.13	**Foot bridge**

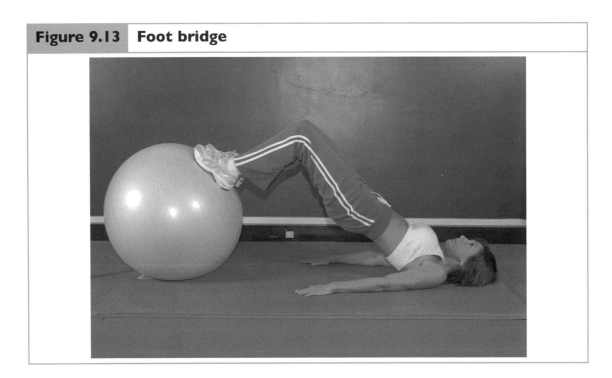

Straight-leg bridge

See Figure 9.14.

Starting position

1. Lie face up on the floor.
2. Place the ball under your feet just below your heels.
3. Keep your feet shoulder-width apart and your arms outstretched.
4. Raise your bottom off the floor until your spine is in the neutral position.
5. There should be a straight line through the knee and hip joint.
6. Only your shoulder blades, head and arms should be resting on the floor.

Action

1. Consciously contract your transversus abdominis.

2. With your feet shoulder-width apart and your arms outstretched, use your feet to roll the ball gently a few inches to one side and then return to the starting point.
3. Repeat, but roll to the opposite side.
4. Repeat five times to each side.
5. Maintain normal breathing throughout.
6. Concentrate on maintaining the starting position during the exercise.

Safety point

Roll only as far as you feel in control of the movement. If you lose control, adopt the starting position and repeat from the point at which you lost control.

Figure 9.14 **Straight-leg bridge**

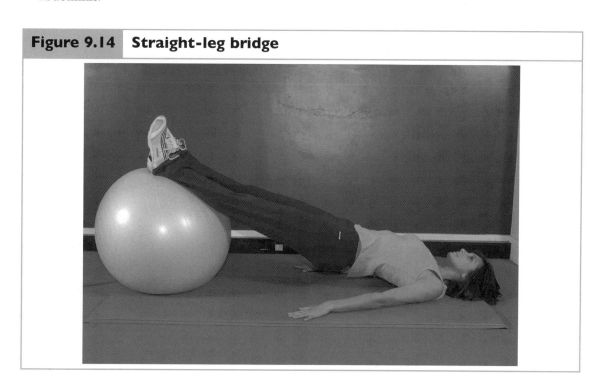

Front bridge

See Figure 9.15.

Starting position

1. Kneel on the floor in front of the ball.
2. Lean forward over the ball so that your chest rests on the ball.
3. Roll over the top of the ball so that your forearms rest on the floor in front of the ball and your pelvis rests directly on top of the ball.
4. Check that your spine is in the neutral position.
5. Keep your neck in neutral by looking down at the floor.
6. Maintain a straight line through your knee, hip and shoulder joints.

Action

1. Consciously contract your transversus abdominis.
2. With your feet together and your forearms on the floor, gently roll the ball a few inches to one side and then return to the start point.
3. Repeat, but roll to the opposite side.
4. Repeat five times to each side.
5. Maintain normal breathing throughout.
6. Concentrate on maintaining the starting position during the exercise.

Safety point

Roll only as far as you feel in control of the movement. Put one foot on the floor if you feel you are about to lose control.

Figure 9.15	**Front bridge**

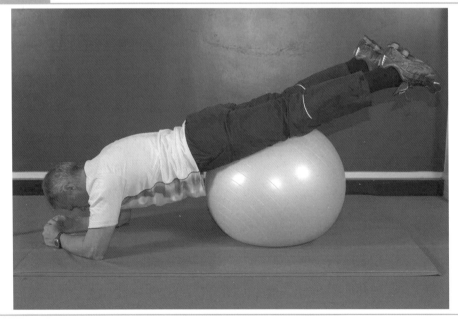

Ab burner

See Figure 9.16.

Starting position

1. Kneel on the floor about 3 feet in front of the ball.
2. Lean forward over the ball so that your forearms rest on the ball.
3. Keep your knees shoulder-width apart.
4. Check that your spine is in the neutral position.
5. Keep your neck in neutral by looking at the floor in front of the ball.

Action

1. Consciously contract your transversus abdominis.

2. With your knees shoulder-width apart and your forearms on the ball, gently roll the ball a few inches to one side and then return to the start point.
3. Repeat, but roll to the opposite side.
4. Repeat five times to each side.
5. Maintain normal breathing throughout.
6. Concentrate on maintaining the starting position during the exercise.

Safety point

Roll only as far as you feel in control of the movement. Use your hands to prevent yourself rolling if you go too far.

Figure 9.16   Ab burner

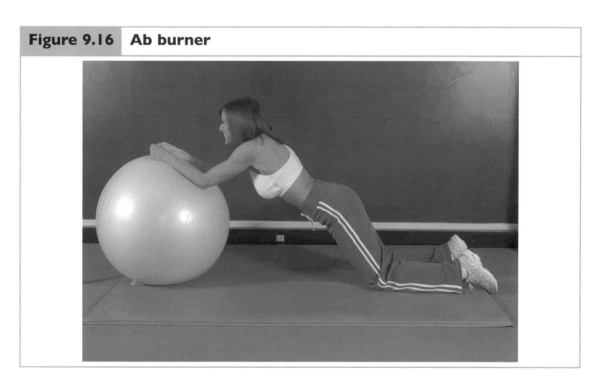

Floor push

See Figures 9.17a and b.

Starting position

1. Kneel on the floor about 3 feet in front of the ball.
2. Lean forward over the ball so that your hands rest on the ball.
3. Keep your knees shoulder-width apart.
4. Check that your spine is in the neutral position.
5. Keep your neck in neutral by looking at the floor in front of the ball.

Action

1. Consciously contract your transversus abdominis.

2. With the knees shoulder-width apart and your hands on the ball, gently lower your body until your chest comes to rest on the ball.
3. Gently raise your body back to the starting point by straightening your arms.
4. Repeat 10 times.
5. Maintain normal breathing throughout.
6. Concentrate on maintaining the starting position during the exercise.

Safety point

Lower your body only as far as feels comfortable.

Figure 9.17   (a) and (b) Floor push

Exercise guidelines

In all new fitness or health programs there is a period known as *habituation* during which the body, in particular the brain, becomes accustomed to the new form of exercise. When the brain becomes accustomed to the exercise, the body will adapt physically in order to accommodate the new level of exercise placed upon it. This period may last for several months. At this stage, the level of exercise can either be increased or maintained, depending on the individual's goals. Many factors influence the speed at which the body becomes accustomed to the new exercise regimen or program, such as frequency, duration, number of repetitions and ability level.

Frequency

Frequency is how often something occurs. In exercise, this is related to the number of times per week that the exercises are carried out. At the start of any new program, at least two sessions per week are recommended in order for the body to adapt to cope with the regularity of the routine. Once the exercises have been carried out regularly for a period of a few weeks, the frequency of sessions can be reduced to once a week in order to maintain the adaptations that the body has made.

Duration

Duration relates to the amount of time spent on each exercise. The actual research carried out in this area is conflicting, and there is no consensus as to the ideal duration of any one exercise. Every individual has a different objective and a different ability level, so it is impossible to recommend a duration period that would benefit all individuals equally. As a

general guide, however, start with an exercise duration of about 15 seconds. If the individual feels capable of increasing the duration, start by adding a period of five seconds to each exercise. If the individual feels that the duration for the exercise is too long, reduce the time of each exercise by five seconds until you reach a suitable duration.

NEED TO KNOW

Core stability training is effective when performed at a comfortable level; the 'no pain, no gain' saying is definitely not recommended in this case.

Repetitions

The number of repetitions simply refers to the number of times the exercise is repeated without a break. As core stability is not a strength issue but relates to a learning process of the brain, the focus is on repeating the exercises at regular intervals to achieve this learning process as quickly as possible. Again, as research is unclear on the ideal number of repetitions, adjust the number of repetitions of each exercise to suit each individual's ability level. Once an individual becomes comfortable with this number of repetitions and feels able to perform more, increase the number until you reach a comfortable level.

NEED TO KNOW

If time is a concern, attempt as many repetitions as you are able. The old saying applies: 'anything is better than nothing.'

EXAMPLE QUESTIONS

9.1 Muscles that provide constant periods of tension in a postural role are otherwise known as what type of muscle?

a) mobilizers

b) global

c) phasic

d) tonic

9.2 Muscles that provide brief periods of tension in a strength role are otherwise known as what type of muscle?

a) stabilizers

b) local

c) phasic

d) tonic

9.3 Which of the following can be considered to be predominantly stabilizing muscles for the core?

a) multifidus, rectus abdominis, diaphragm

b) multifidus, transversus abdominis, diaphragm

c) pelvic floor, rectus abdominis, diaphragm

d) multifidus, erector spinae, diaphragm

9.4 Which of the following can be considered to be predominantly mobilizing muscles for the core?

a) multifidus, rectus abdominis, diaphragm

b) multifidus, transversus abdominis, diaphragm

c) erector spinae, rectus abdominis, external obliques

d) multifidus, erector spinae, diaphragm

9.5 Which of the following can be considered to be predominantly a stabilizing muscle for the hip joint?

a) external obliques

b) gluteus maximus

c) gluteus minimus

d) gluteus medius

EXAMPLE QUESTIONS cont.

9.6 Which of the following can be considered to be predominantly a mobilizing muscle for the hip joint?

a) internal obliques

b) gluteus maximus

c) transversus abdominis

d) gluteus medius

9.7 When local muscles contract to compress the 'fluid ball' in the abdomen it is known as what?

a) neutral spine or zone

b) intra-abdominal pressure

c) hydraulic amplifier effect

d) thoracolumbar fascia gain

9.8 An increase in the tension of the connective tissues in the spinal region is known as what?

a) neutral spine or zone

b) intra-abdominal pressure

c) fluid ball pressure

d) thoracolumbar fascia gain

9.9 Research has suggested that what minimum percentage of maximum contraction is sufficient to create sufficient intra-abdominal pressure to stabilize the spine?

a) 70

b) 100

c) 50

d) 30

9.10 What best relates to the following statement – '*when there is minimal force placed on the spine and the structures that surround it such as tendons, cartilage and ligaments.*'?

a) anterior pelvic tilt

b) neutral zone

c) intra-abdominal pressure

d) thoracolumbar fascia gain

EXAMPLE QUESTIONS cont.

9.11 True or false? Normal screening procedures should be carried out prior to prescribing core stabilization exercises, but those with back problems should be excluded.

True ☐   False ☐

9.12 The length of time, number of repetitions and frequency of practice of conscious contraction required to develop subconscious contraction control of the transversus abdominis can take up to how long?

a) a few hours
b) a few days
c) a few weeks
d) a few months

Further reading

Abrahams, P., Craven, J. and Lumley, J. (2005) *Illustrated Clinical Anatomy*, Hodder Arnold

Norris, C.M. (2001) *Abdominal Training* (2nd ed.), A & C Black

Richardson, C., Jull, G., Hodges, P. and Hides, J. (2003) *Therapeutic Exercise for Spinal Segmental Stabilization in Low Back Pain*, Churchill Livingstone

Sewell, D., Watkins, P. and Griffin, M. (2005) *Sport and Exercise Science: An Introduction*, Hodder Arnold

Tortora, G.J. and Grabowski, S.R. (2003) *Principles of Anatomy & Physiology* (10th ed.), Wiley

Wilson, K.J.W. and Waugh, A. (1998) *Ross and Wilson Anatomy and Physiology in Health and Illness*, Churchill Livingstone

NOTES

COMPONENTS AND PRINCIPLES OF FITNESS

OBJECTIVES

After completing this chapter, you will be able to

1 Define the terms 'physical fitness,' 'wellness' and 'health-related fitness.'

2 Define the term 'hypokinetic disease.'

3 List and describe the components of fitness.

4 State the American College of Sports Medicine (ACSM) guidelines relating to the components of fitness.

5 Describe how components of fitness can affect the body.

6 Explain the factors affecting physical fitness.

7 List and describe the principles of fitness.

Instructing Exercise and Fitness Knowledge

Basic Anatomy and Physiology

- The application of the principles and variables of fitness to the components of fitness.

- How to apply the principles and variables of fitness to a range of activities that will achieve various health benefits and the required fitness development.

Instructing Physical Activity and Exercise Knowledge

Components of fitness

- Definitions of fitness:
  - Physical fitness
  - Health-related fitness
  - Wellness

- Components of fitness and how they can be assessed:
  - Aerobic capacity
  - Muscular strength
  - Muscular resistance
  - Flexibility
  - Body composition

- Principles of fitness, including FITT, overload, specificity, reversibility
- ACSM guidelines for developing each component of fitness
- Methods of flexibility training (static, ballistic, dynamic, PNF, CRAC)

Introduction

This chapter deals with the components and principles of fitness. Instructors should be able to identify the components and principles of fitness and list the guidelines associated with these.

Later chapters in the book provide information regarding the practical application of theoretical knowledge, which, along with the content covered in this chapter, will provide you with the understanding and ability to design appropriate exercise programs for apparently healthy individuals in line with current guidelines for exercise.

Definitions of fitness

There are many definitions and individual perceptions of 'fitness.' For some, fitness might include the ability to perform some activity at a competitive level, whereas to others it might be the ability to perform everyday tasks without undue stress and fatigue. Fitness might also include a health or wellness component, which can relate to the absence of disease.

Health-related physical fitness

The American College of Sports Medicine (ACSM) defines health-related physical fitness as 'an ability to perform daily activities with vigor and the demonstration of traits and capacities that are associated with a low risk of premature development of hypokinetic diseases.'

The closest translation for the word *hypokinetic* is 'low movement.' Hypokinetic diseases are associated with low levels of activity, such as heart disease, obesity and high blood pressure. For the purpose of this book, it is assumed that any prescribed exercise, regardless of the definition of fitness, will be beneficial in reducing the risk of hypokinetic disease.

Wellness

The ACSM definition of health-related physical fitness relates only to physical well-being, not to psychological well-being. However, there are many advocates of the notion that exercise can have a positive psychological effect, for example promoting mental, social and emotional well-being. The World Health Organization (WHO) promotes the idea of *wellness*, defining it as 'a state of complete physical, mental and social well-being, and not merely the absence of disease or infirmity.'

Physical fitness

Although the terms health-related physical fitness and wellness can be defined clearly, the most common anecdotal term used within the health and fitness industry is *fitness*. The ACSM distinguishes between health-related physical fitness and physical fitness, defining the latter as 'a set of attributes that relates to the ability to perform physical activity.'

Components of physical fitness

Fitness, or to be more precise physical fitness, can be divided into discreet components that can be trained or adapted individually. Depending on the type of training carried out, an individual can be classed as 'fit' in one or more of the individual components.

The ACSM lists the following components of health-related physical fitness: *cardiovascular endurance*, *muscular strength*, *muscular endurance*, *body composition* and *flexibility*. The components of physical fitness are the same but also include *motor skills*, which comprise several subcomponents. This book focuses on the components of health-related physical fitness.

Cardiovascular endurance

Cardiovascular endurance is the ability of the heart and lungs to deliver oxygen to the working muscles (sometimes known as *aerobic capacity*) and for the muscles to use this oxygen to generate work.

Measuring cardiovascular endurance

Cardiovascular endurance is often measured as *volume of oxygen* (VO_2), with VO_{2max} being the maximum amount of oxygen that can be delivered to the working muscles. The units used to measure VO_2 are milliliters of oxygen per kilogram bodyweight per minute ($mLO_2.kg^{-1}.min^{-1}$).

How to improve cardiovascular endurance

The best types of exercise for improving cardiovascular endurance are those that involve the use of large muscle groups over a prolonged period of time at an intensity that is classed as aerobic (for example walking, hiking, running, stepping, swimming, cycling, dancing, skiing, skipping and so on). As the intensity of the exercise increases, the amount of oxygen required to cope with the demands made by the muscles increases; therefore, the heart rate increases in proportion. This increase in heart rate due to an increase in exercise intensity is known as a *linear relationship*. In other words, there is an equal increase in heart rate for an equal increase in intensity. Figure 10.1 shows that after performing regular cardiovascular exercise for a period of time, the same intensity can usually be maintained with a lower heart rate.

FITT guidelines for cardiovascular training

It can be difficult to know the correct duration and intensity of exercise to recommend in order for your clients to achieve optimum

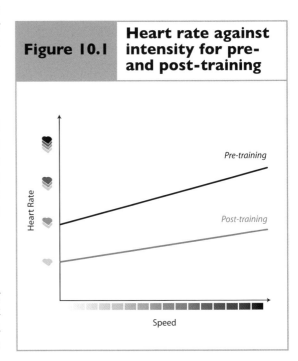

Figure 10.1 **Heart rate against intensity for pre- and post-training**

benefits in terms of cardiovascular endurance. Too little exercise might not have the desired effect, whereas too much might result in a condition known as *overtraining,* where damage to the body may occur in the form of an injury or a respiratory disease such as the common cold. For this reason, the ACSM has developed guidelines known as the *FITT principles.* FITT stands for *frequency, intensity, time* and *type.* Table 10.1 outlines the FITT guidelines for cardiovascular training.

Some clients may not be able to achieve 20 minutes of cardiovascular exercise or maintain intensities above 55 percent of maximum heart rate. Therefore, the guidelines should be used to set targets for clients, rather than being absolute goals that clients must achieve. Any progressions should be limited to an increase of no more than 20 percent of duration each week until clients can exercise at a moderate to vigorous intensity for 20–60 minutes. Increases in duration and frequency usually precede intensity increases.

Benefits of cardiovascular endurance

There are many benefits associated with an increase in cardiovascular endurance. One of the most important is a reduced risk in coronary artery disease; other benefits include the followng:

- Reduced blood pressure
- Reduced body fat
- Lower heart rate for given intensity of exercise
- Increased exercise threshold for accumulation of blood lactate (the performer can exercise at a higher intensity before lactic acid builds up to the point at which intensity has to be reduced)
- Increase in high-density-lipoprotein (good) cholesterol

Muscular strength

Muscular strength is the maximum amount of force that a muscle or muscle group can generate.

Measuring muscular strength

Both static and dynamic muscular strength can be measured. In static strength testing, machines called dynamometers measure how much force an individual can exert against it without any movement. In dynamic strength testing, an individual moves an external load (usually free weights or resistance machines). This is known as *1 repetition max* testing or *1RM* testing, where the maximum amount of weight that can be lifted once with good form is recorded. It is possible to predict 1RM from multiple RM testing, for example 6RM is the maximum amount of weight that can be lifted six times, which can then be used to predict IRM.

Table 10.1	FITT guidelines for cardiovascular training
Frequency	3–5 days per week
Intensity	55–90 percent of maximum heart rate* (RPE 12–16: see pages 219–20)
Time	20–60 minutes continuous or intermittent aerobic exercise
Type	Involving large muscle mass; rhythmic; aerobic
Key: RPE = rate of perceived exertion; *Maximum heart rate is calculated as 220 minus age.	

How to improve muscular strength

Muscular strength can be developed through resistance training, including using machine and free weights, body weight and resistance bands. Developing muscular strength normally requires relatively high resistance (or weight) and few repetitions, and is usually associated with an increase in muscle size. Because of the intense nature of this type of training, it is common for individuals to experience pain or stiffness in the muscles that have been trained in the days following a training session. This sensation is known as delayed-onset muscle soreness or DOMS (see page 41).

Muscular endurance

Muscular endurance is the ability of a muscle or muscle group to perform repeated contractions against a resistance over a period of time and is associated with resistance training using relatively low intensity and high repetitions. Hypertrophy is not usually associated with this type of training, although DOMS can be experienced if training is carried out to fatigue. Testing normally involves recording the maximum number of repetitions of a task, such as a push-up or sit-up, that can be achieved.

Benefits of resistance training

There are many benefits of resistance training that vary slightly depending on the type of training. The benefits include the following:

- Increase in muscle mass, which increases resting metabolic rate
- Increase in bone mass
- Reduced risk of osteoporosis
- Increased glucose tolerance
- Increase in joint integrity
- Improved posture

- Reduction in back pain
- Reduced risk of hypertension
- Reduced risk of diabetes

The benefits of muscular endurance training are similar to those of muscular strength training, but with less emphasis on increased muscle mass and more emphasis on muscle tone. One of the long-term effects of resistance training is hypertrophy, or an increase in the size of the muscle being trained. This usually occurs after the first few weeks of training as strength gains in the first few weeks are as a result of 'learning' mechanisms known as *neural* changes.

DOMS can occur a day or two after a particularly intense training session. Light aerobic exercise following resistance training can reduce this effect.

FITT guidelines for resistance training

Table 10.2 outlines the FITT guidelines for resistance training.

Note: ACSM guidelines recommend a timing sequence of three seconds concentric and three seconds eccentric contraction for all resistance exercises that involve a full range of motion.

Volitional fatigue is the point at which the individual performing the exercise thinks that he or she can no longer carry on. This can be uncomfortable for the performer, so to encourage adherence to an exercise program it is sensible to adopt a flexible approach to this guideline for individuals who are not familiar with exercising to fatigue levels.

Flexibility

Flexibility is the ability to move a joint through its complete range of motion.

Table 10.2	FITT principles for resistance training	
Frequency	2–3 nonconsecutive sessions per week	
Intensity	1 set of 3–20 repetitions to volitional fatigue while maintaining good form (RPE 16–20)	
Time	Enough to carry out 8–10 separate exercises for total body	
Type	Body weight; machines; free weights; bands	
Key: RPE = rate of perceived exertion		

Testing flexibility

Flexibility is joint specific in that an individual may be flexible in one joint and not in another. Therefore, there is no one test that is whole-body specific, and all joints must be assessed individually using *goniometry*, where the angle of each joint is measured and compared against tables for normal ranges of motion. A common flexibility test used in the health and fitness industry is the 'sit and reach' test, where an individual sits with straight legs and reaches forward to record the distance reached with the fingertips. This measures only hamstring and lower back flexibility.

Benefits of flexibility

One of the main benefits of maintaining the range of motion within joints is that it allows individuals to carry out daily activities as long as possible throughout their lives. Although it is frequently recommended that stretching can help prevent injury, there is little evidence to support the notion: it has been shown that a high degree as well as a low degree of flexibility can increase injury risk. It is recommended that people with tight muscles would probably benefit most from static stretching, whereas people who are naturally supple should not engage in more than light stretching. The most effective stretching occurs when the muscles are warm.

Types of stretching

There are many types of stretching exercises, including *static*, *dynamic*, *PNF* and *ballistic*. Below is a simple description of the common types of stretches.

Static stretching

A static stretch is held for a period of time at a point of mild tension. The point of tension is usually the point at which the stretch reflex is invoked. If the stretch is held for long enough, the tension usually subsides and the stretch can be taken further if required. If a partner or another group of muscles assists in the stretching process, it is known as an *active* stretch. If there is no assistance, it is a *passive* stretch. Research on the optimum time period for a stretch is vague, but guidelines relating to the recommended time period are shown in Table 10.3.

Dynamic stretching

A dynamic stretch refers to stretching in motion where an agonist muscle is contracted to stretch an antagonist muscle. This type of stretching is usually carried out in a slow and controlled manner in order to minimize the risk of injury and to mimic the types of movement that may be used in the exercises to follow.

Ballistic stretching

Ballistic stretches are bouncing movements caused by momentum or gravity. This type of stretching is usually carried out only by athletes who are familiar with this type of stretching: as there is little control of the movement, there is a greater risk of injury than with other types of stretching.

PNF stretching

PNF stands for proprioceptive neuromuscular facilitation. This is a type of partner-assisted stretching that is normally used for tight or injured muscles. This type of stretching requires training, so it should be performed only by those who are qualified to do so. *CRAC* (contraction relax antagonist contract) is another form of this type of stretching. Table 10.3 outlines the FITT guidelines for flexibility training.

Body composition

Body composition refers to the ratio of fat to lean tissue in an individual: in other words, how lean, overweight or obese a person is. Even though body composition is listed as a component of fitness, it is probably more accurate to associate it with an indication of health as excess body fat is associated with hypertension, diabetes, stroke, coronary heart disease and hyperlipidemia. Body composition is also affected greatly by other components of fitness, such as cardiovascular and resistance training.

Measuring body composition

Body composition can be measured in many different ways, including body mass index (BMI), using skinfolds, underwater weighing and electrical impedance methods. Some methods are more accurate than others. One of the easiest methods is BMI. Although this is not a direct measurement of body fat percentage, it does give an indication of overweight or obesity, which has been defined by the ACSM as the percentage of body fat at which an individual's risk of disease increases. BMI is calculated using the following equation:

$$BMI = \frac{Weight \ (kg)}{Height^2 \ (m^2)}$$

Table 10.4 shows how BMI is used to classify body composition.

Although the causes of obesity can include hypothalamic, endocrine and genetic disorders, diet and physical inactivity are the prime factors. It is generally accepted and recommended by the ACSM that an increase in calorie expenditure and a decrease in calorie intake are the most effective long-term methods for treating obesity: between 150 and 400 kcal of daily

Table 10.3	FITT guidelines for flexibility training
Frequency	Minimum 2–3 sessions per week; ideally 5–7 sessions per week
Intensity	To the end range of motion at a point of tightness, without pain
Time	15–30 seconds, 2–4 times per stretch
Type	Static, preceded by a warm-up

Table 10.4	BMI classifications
BMI	Classification
<25	Normal
25–30	Overweight
>30	Obese

energy expenditure is recommended for weight-loss programs.

Motor skills

Many subcomponents are associated with motor skills, including speed, power, agility, coordination and balance. All of these areas can be improved with training.

Speed

Speed is the ability to move quickly from one point to another and can be improved through muscle coordination, efficient body movement, core strength and flexibility.

Power

Power is a combination of strength and speed and can be developed through plyometric and resistance training.

Agility

Agility is the ability to change direction with speed.

Balance

Balance is the ability to maintain equilibrium at all times. Proprioceptors in the body give information to the brain on the position of all limbs, as well as balance information from the inner ear and the eyes.

Coordination

Coordination is the ability to move the limbs precisely in a particular direction.

There are many theories regarding the storage of movement patterns, known as motor programs. One theory proposed by Schmidt (2003) suggests that typical movements such as bending and squatting are stored with related information such as muscle timing and velocities. All other movements are just adaptations of these typical stored movements. For example, the movement sequence for a jump is similar to that of a squat because of the relationship of the body segments. A jump sequence, however, is entirely different from that of a leg press or leg extension. There are no recommended guidelines for motor skills in relation to FITT principles.

TASK

List and briefly describe the components of fitness and state the recommended guidelines related to each component.

Factors influencing physical fitness

When training for any of the components of fitness, various factors may influence the outcome of the type of training. These factors include *body type, gender, fitness level, lifestyle* and *age*.

Body type

The distribution of fiber type within muscles is determined at birth. A person with a higher percentage distribution of fast-twitch fibers will be more predisposed to strength-type events, whereas a person with a high percentage of slow-twitch fibers will be predisposed to endurance-type events.

There are three extreme classifications of body type that can be used to describe the overall shape of an individual: *endomorph, ectomorph* and *mesomorph* (see Table 10.5). It is common for individuals to be a combination of more than one type, so a grading system for each classification can be used.

Gender

Gender relates simply to either male or female. This has some implications on the components of fitness. For example, cardiovascular potential (VO_{2max}) is typically 15–30 percent lower in females than in males. Men are also capable of greater muscle hypertrophy as a result of strength training as they tend to have a greater proportion of fast-twitch fibers.

Table 10.5	Characteristics of different body types
Endomorph	• A pear-shaped body • A rounded head • Wide hips and shoulders • Wider front to back rather than side to side • A lot of fat on the body, upper arms and thighs
Ectomorph	• A high forehead • A receding chin • Narrow shoulders and hips • A narrow chest and abdomen • Thin arms and legs • Little muscle and fat
Mesomorph	• A wedge-shaped body • A cubical head • Wide, broad shoulders • Muscled arms and legs • Narrow hips • Narrow from front to back rather than side to side

Fitness

A less fit individual will initially make greater improvements in components of fitness than a fitter person. This should be taken into account when setting goals and targets with clients (see Chapter 12).

Lifestyle

There are many aspects of lifestyle that can affect components of fitness. One of the main aspects is psychological stress, which can have a detrimental effect on the way in which individuals train. Smoking and drinking alcohol can have a similar effect.

Age

Aging can decrease the individual components of fitness, but with a regular training routine these diminishing effects can be minimized and in some cases reversed. For example flexibility can very quickly be lost, but many older individuals retain flexibility by participating in exercises such as yoga.

TASK

Describe how various factors can influence physical fitness.

Principles of fitness

When designing any exercise program it is important to remember certain fundamental factors that can have an affect on the outcome of the program. These factors are called *principles of fitness.* These principles must be taken into account with all individuals in relation to the design of a training or exercise program.

Lifestyle

The body can adapt to the demands of various types of exercise, and the type of adaptation that takes place is dependent on the muscle fibers involved and the types of exercise. For example, type 1 fibers will adapt to endurance training, whereas type 2 fibers will adapt to more intense strength training.

Adaptation

This principle states that the adaptations derived from an exercise are specific to the exercise and to the muscles involved in that exercise. For example, runners show little improvement in the muscular endurance of their arm muscles, whereas cyclists show most of their muscular endurance improvement in their leg muscles.

Overload

In order for an individual to adapt to a new demand or routine, *overload* must be achieved. Overload can be described as 'taking the body or system to a point just beyond what it is usually accustomed to' (ACSM, 2006). If any system within the body (a muscle or an organ) is made to work harder than it normally does on a regular basis, it will undergo certain physical changes to adapt to the new workload. It is important to remember that the body should be taken to a workload just beyond normal levels; if it is taken too far, injury may occur.

Progressive overload

If the workload of a training program is not progressed, the individual will not continue to adapt. Instead, once the body has adapted to the current workload, it will not attempt to adapt any further. In order to progress, the workload must be periodically changed once the body has become accustomed to the previous workload. The rate of progression is specific to each individual and can also be affected by various factors:

Fitness level

Less fit individuals will progress at a faster rate than fitter individuals.

Experience

An individual with past experience of certain exercises will progress at a faster rate than those with no experience.

Injury

An injury to a specific site can reverse any gains previously made at that site. It is important to remember that the rest of the body may be trained to prevent total body reversibility.

Environment

The nature of the environment can affect progression in several ways. For example, altitude training can have an effect on oxygen transport, whereas heat and cold can affect the rate of progression.

Reversibility

Just as the body can become stronger if the workload is increased, the body can become weaker over a period of time if the workload is reduced. It is possible for specific fitness components to diminish within two weeks of cessation of exercise. This principle is known as *reversibility*.

As all individuals progress at different rates, it is important that the frequency, intensity and duration of exercise are manipulated to suit the individual. In any health-related fitness program, individuals should be encouraged to start slowly and begin at levels that can easily be maintained. Progression should then be encouraged when the individual feels that he or she can cope with the current workload and is able to progress. There are many ways in which overload can be achieved within a program in order to progress to achieve adaptation. Lever length, speed, resistance and gravity are among many variables in which to progress a program of exercise.

TASK

List and briefly explain the principles used in prescribing exercise.

EXAMPLE QUESTIONS

10.1 The ACSM defines what as '*an ability to perform daily activities with vigor and the demonstration of traits and capacities that are associated with a low risk of premature development of hypokinetic diseases*'?
   a) wellness
   b) physical fitness
   c) health-related physical fitness
   d) mental health

10.2 The World Health Organization defines what as '*a state of complete physical, mental and social well-being and not merely the absence of disease or infirmity*'?
   a) wellness
   b) physical fitness
   c) health-related fitness
   d) mental health

10.3 The ACSM defines what as '*a set of attributes that people have or achieve that relates to the ability to perform physical activity*'?
   a) wellness
   b) physical fitness
   c) health-related fitness
   d) mental health

10.4 VO_{2max} is measured in what?
   a) $mmolO_2.kg^{-1}min^{-1}$
   b) $mlCO_2.kg^{-1}min^{-1}$
   c) $mlO_2.kg^{-1}min^{-1}$
   d) $l.kg^{-1}min^{-1}$

10.5 An increase in intensity that results in an equal increase in heart rate has what kind of relationship?
   a) linear
   b) nonlinear
   c) exponential
   d) inverse-exponential

EXAMPLE QUESTIONS cont.

10.6 What is the term used to define an increase in muscle cross section?
a) DOMS
b) atrophy
c) hypertrophy
d) tone

10.7 What is the term used to define a decrease in muscle cross section?
a) DOMS
b) atrophy
c) hypertrophy
d) tone

10.8 What is the term used to describe the perception of soreness in a muscle in the period shortly following intense exercise training?
a) DOMS
b) atrophy
c) hypertrophy
d) tone

10.9 The type of stretching that involves the use of a partner is known as what?
a) static
b) ballistic
c) dynamic
d) PNF

10.10 The type of stretching that predominantly involves the use of momentum and gravity is known as what?
a) static
b) ballistic
c) dynamic
d) PNF

EXAMPLE QUESTIONS cont.

10.11 Which of the following formulae can be used to calculate BMI?
   a) $weight^2/height$
   b) $weight/height^2$
   c) $height/weight^2$
   d) $height^2/weight$

10.12 In relation to BMI, what figure is classed as obese?
   a) over 25
   b) over 30
   c) over 20
   d) over 15

Further reading

American College of Sports Medicine (2006) *ACSM Guidelines to Exercise Testing and Prescription* (7th ed.), Lippincott, Williams & Wilkins

Baechle, R.T. (2000) *Essentials of Strength Training and Conditioning*, Human Kinetics

Bompa, T.O. (1999) *Periodisation Training for Sports*, Human Kinetics

Bouchard, C., Shepard, R. and Stephens, T. (1994) *Physical Activity, Fitness and Health*, Human Kinetics

Howley, E.T. and Franks, B.D. (1997) *Health Fitness Instructor's Handbook* (3rd ed.) Human Kinetics

Marieb, E. (1998) *Human Anatomy and Physiology* (4th ed.) The Benjamin Cummings Publishing Company Inc.

McArdle, W.D., Katch, F.I. and Katch, V.L. (1996) *Exercise Physiology*, Lippincott, Williams & Wilkins

Schmidt, R.A, (2003) Motor schema theory after 27 years: *Research Quarterly for Exercise and Sport.* Dec; 74(4):366–75

Sewell, D., Watkins, P. and Griffin, M. (2005) *Sport and Exercise Science: An Introduction*, Hodder Arnold

Tortora, G.J. and Grabowski, S.R. (2003) *Principles of Anatomy and Physiology* (10th ed.), Wiley

Wilmore, J.H. and Costhill, D.L. (2004) *Physiology of Sport and Exercise* (3rd ed.), Human Kinetics

Wilson, K.J.W. and Waugh, A. (1998) *Ross and Wilson Anatomy and Physiology in Health and Illness*, Churchill Livingstone

NOTES

PRACTICAL APPLICATION OF HEALTH AND FITNESS

PART TWO

Part 2 looks at practical methods of applying the theory covered in Part 1. There is also a list of recommended reading for each chapter, should you wish to gain more in-depth knowledge of a particular subject area.

SCREENING FOR EXERCISE AND SAFETY ISSUES

OBJECTIVES

After completing this chapter, you will be able to

1   Define the term 'screening' in relation to the health and fitness industry.

2   List and describe the different types of screening questionnaire available for the health and fitness industry.

3   Explain the term 'risk stratification' and list the coronary artery risk factors identified by the American College of Sports Medicine.

4   Describe general issues relating to facility equipment management.

5   Describe procedures of risk assessment prior to exercise sessions.

6   Explain the procedure for dealing with an emergency situation during an exercise session.

Instructing Exercise and Fitness Knowledge

Basic Anatomy and Physiology

- The importance of careful and thorough planning and preparation for sessions.

- The requirements for health and safety that are relevant to the activities you are planning, for example factors that affect group/individual working space, your organization's health and safety policies and procedures.

- The factors that affect the ability to exercise; the screening process, including primary and secondary risk factors of coronary heart disease.

- The Exercise and Fitness Code of Ethical Practice.

- Reasons for temporary deferral of exercise; referral; informed consent.

- The emergency procedures of the facility/organization.

- The Physical Activity Readiness Questionnaire (PAR-Q) and how to record information on it.

- How to identify and agree upon objectives for the session based upon collected information.

- Manufacturers' and organizations' guidelines for replacement of equipment.
- The safe storage of free-weight equipment.
- What to look for when checking equipment.
- The health and environmental factors that can influence safety; factors that affect group/individual working space.

Instructing Physical Activity and Exercise Knowledge

Components of Fitness
- Coronary heart disease risk factors

Introduction

This chapter deals with various screening methods used within the health and fitness industry. Instructors should be able to identify safety issues and describe methods of screening and the guidelines associated with these.

Later chapters in the book provide the knowledge required in relation to program design, which, along with the content covered in this chapter, will provide you with the understanding and ability to design appropriate exercise programs for apparently healthy individuals, in line with current guidelines for exercise.

Screening for exercise

One of the most important roles of a health and fitness instructor is to help individuals determine their current health and fitness status prior to undertaking a program of exercise. This can aid you not only in planning and designing a safe and effective program but also in identifying any professional medical guidance that may be needed before the individual starts a program.

The process of determining the health and fitness status of an individual is known as *health screening*, normally shortened to *screening*. In a health and fitness environment, two methods of screening are available to the instructor. One method involves the use of pre-exercise questionnaires, of which there are many types, and the other involves verbal methods.

Pre-exercise questionnaires

Health screening questionnaires

Many types of pre-exercise health questionnaires are available, the most common in the health and fitness industry being the *Physical Activity Readiness Questionnaire*, or *PAR-Q* (see Figure 11.1 for an example). Developed by the Canadian Society for Exercise Physiology, the PAR-Q is a short questionnaire that can help to identify possible symptoms of cardiovascular, pulmonary and metabolic disease, as well as other conditions that might be aggravated by exercise. The form is self-explanatory and brief: if any conditions are identified, the form advises the individual to seek medical approval prior to undertaking a program of exercise. If no conditions are identified, the form encourages a program of light to moderate exercise to be undertaken at an intensity relevant to the current fitness level of the individual.

PAR-Q forms should be given out to all individuals and completed prior to the start of an exercise program. The form should then be interpreted by a suitably qualified professional and dealt with in a confidential manner. If the instructor feels that the form reveals anything that is beyond the capacity of their training or experience, they should refer the case to a suitably qualified colleague or supervisor.

Figure 11.1   **Example of a PAR-Q**

PAR-Q and You

Please read the following questions and answer each one honestly.

	Yes	No
1. Has your doctor ever said that you have a heart condition and that you should only do physical activity recommended by a doctor?	—	—
2. Do you feel pain in your chest when you do physical activity?	—	—
3. In the past month, have you had chest pain while you were not doing physical activity?	—	—
4. Do you lose your balance because of dizziness or do you ever lose consciousness?	—	—
5. Do you have a bone or joint problem that could be made worse by physical activity?	—	—
6. Is your doctor currently prescribing drugs for your blood pressure or heart condition?	—	—
7. Do you know of any other reason why you should *not* do physical activity?	—	—

If you answered YES to one or more questions:

Talk to your doctor **BEFORE** you become more physically active or have a fitness appraisal. Discuss with your doctor which kinds of activities you wish to participate in.

If you answered NO to all questions:

You can be reasonably sure that you can:

- Start becoming much more physically active. Start slowly and build up gradually.
- Take part in a fitness appraisal. This is a good way to determine your basic fitness level. It is recommended that you have your blood pressure evaluated.

Figure 11.1	**Example of a PAR-Q cont.**

However, delay becoming active if:

- You are not feeling well because of temporary illness such as a cold or 'flu.
- You are or may be pregnant: talk to your doctor first.

Please note: *If your health changes so that you then answer YES to any of the above questions, tell your fitness or health professional. Ask whether you should change your physical activity plan.*

'I have read, understood and completed this questionnaire. Any questions I had were answered to my full satisfaction.'

Name: _____

Signature: _____

Date: _____

Signature of witness: _____

Signature of parent/guardian: _____

Note: This physical activity clearance is valid for a maximum of 12 months from the date it is completed, and becomes invalid if your condition changes so that you would answer YES to any of the seven questions.

Source: Physical Activity Readiness Questionnaire (PAR-Q) 2002. Reprinted with permission from the Canadian Society for Exercise Physiology.

Physical activity screening questionnaires

Prior to designing a program of exercise for an individual, it is recommended that previous and current client fitness levels are established. One of the methods commonly employed within the health and fitness industry is a *physical activity screening questionnaire*, which is often used to ensure the exercise program is at the optimum level for the client. However, a fitness questionnaire is not a replacement for the PAR-Q but rather a supplement to it.

There is no accepted standard of fitness questionnaire available, and many different types are used within the health and fitness industry. Typical questionnaires include the following questions:

1. Do you currently participate in any form of exercise?
2. How often do you participate in exercise?
3. What types of exercise do you currently participate in?
4. How long do you normally exercise for during each session?
5. Would you class your exercise as moderate or vigorous?
6. Can you walk briskly for 30 minutes without fatigue?
7. Can you jog for 20 minutes without fatigue?
8. What types of exercises do you enjoy doing?
9. What types of exercise do you not like doing?
10. If you do not currently exercise, when was the last time you participated in regular exercise?
11. How often did you participate in regular exercise and what type of exercise was it?

As with all information of a personal nature, the physical activity screening questionnaire must be treated confidentially. Confidentiality and other such values are explained in more detail within a set of standards known as the Code of Ethics. This applies to instructors within the health and fitness industry and constitutes a set of guidelines within which to work.

Lifestyle questionnaires

Lifestyle questionnaires are also commonly used in the health and fitness industry to elicit information about diet, exercise and activities regarded as *lifestyle activities*, such as walking, housework and gardening. Lifestyle activities have been shown to have numerous health benefits and can be integrated into a typical daily lifestyle for most individuals, and these types of questionnaires can help instructors to identify areas of lifestyle that could be improved and could be incorporated into an overall program of exercise.

As with physical activity screening questionnaires, lifestyle questionnaires are not a replacement for the PAR-Q but a supplement to it. Many lifestyle questionnaires are in use in the health and fitness industry, but typical questionnaires include the following questions:

1. Do you currently smoke and, if so, how much?
2. Do you drink alcohol and, if so, how much on average each week?
3. Do you work at a desk each day?
4. How do you travel to work?
5. What do you do at break times?
6. Are there any stairs at your place of work?
7. What is your typical daily routine?
8. How far do you walk on a typical day?
9. Would you consider yourself to have a healthy diet?
10. Do you snack between meals?
11. When do you have your last meal of the day?

Note: With all pre-exercise questionnaires, the instructor must respect the confidentiality of all written material relating to client information by ensuring safe storage and private access.

Verbal screening

In addition to the PAR-Q screening form, instructors can screen clients verbally prior to an exercise session. A certain amount of time may have elapsed between a client completing a PAR-Q and actually beginning a program of exercise. Within this period of time injuries may have occurred, so individuals should be asked if they know of any reason why they should not exercise or if they have any current injury that could prevent them from exercising. In certain facilities, it is also possible for members to access studio classes without going through the screening process. For this reason, when supervising a one-to-one or group exercise session it is advisable to carry out verbal screening prior to the start of the session.

It is at the instructor's discretion to decide whether any response warrants medical referral. All general practitioner offices have their own procedure for exercise referral, so it is important to be aware of the procedures employed at geographically relevant offices. Verbal screening is also confidential; therefore, discretion must be used in a group exercise situation.

Note: Some health and fitness facilities use an informed consent form that individuals agree to and sign before undertaking an exercise program. These forms state the benefits and risks associated with exercise and are intended as a precaution against liability.

TASK

List the types of screening available to instructors and describe the benefits of each.

Risk stratification

Although the PAR-Q screening process is considered an acceptable level of screening within the health and fitness industry, many other more in-depth health screening questionnaires can be used. These questionnaires can provide a more detailed medical and lifestyle history.

One such questionnaire is the American Heart Association (AHA)/American College of Sports Medicine (ACSM) Health/Fitness Facility Preparticipation Screening Questionnaire (see Figure 11.2), which can identify a broad range of diseases that can be aggravated by exercise. It can also help to identify certain conditions that have been shown to increase the risk of heart disease, known as coronary artery disease risk factors. The ACSM identifies the following as coronary artery disease risk factors:

1. **Family history:** myocardial infarction or sudden death before age 55 in father, brother or son; before age 65 in mother, sister or daughter.
2. **Smoking:** current smoker or quit within previous six months.
3. **Hypertension:** systolic blood pressure of 140 mmHg or above, or diastolic of 90 mmHg or above, on at least two occasions.
4. **Dyslipidemia:** total serum cholesterol of more than 5.2 mmol/l, or low-density lipoprotein (LDL) more than 3.4 mmol/l, or high-density lipoprotein (HDL) less than 1.03 mmol/l.
5. **Obesity:** body mass index (BMI) of 30 kg/m^2 or above.
6. **Sedentary lifestyle:** not participating in regular exercise.
7. **Impaired fasting glucose:** 100 mg/dl or more.

Figure 11.2	Example of a risk stratification questionnaire	

Mark all true statements

History – You have had
___ a heart attack
___ heart surgery
___ cardiac catheterization
___ coronary angioplasty
___ a pacemaker
___ defibrillator
___ heart valve disease
___ heart failure
___ a heart transplant
___ heart disease

Symptoms – You experience
___ chest pain with exertion
___ unreasonable breathlessness
___ dizziness or fainting
___ heart medication

Other issues:
___ you have diabetes
___ you have asthma or COPD
___ you get a burning sensation in the legs when walking short distances
___ you have musculoskeletal problems that limit physical activity
___ you have concerns about exercise safety
___ you take prescribed drugs
___ you are pregnant

Risk factors:
___ you are a male over 45 years old
___ you are female over 55 years old
___ you smoke or quit within the last six months
___ your blood pressure is above 140/90 mmHg
___ your total cholesterol is above 5.2 mmol/l
___ you have heart attack or sudden death in the family (male before 55 years, female before 65 years)
___ you are sedentary
___ you are classed as obese

If you marked any of the statements in this section as true, consult your GP before taking part in an exercise program.

___ none of the above

You can exercise.

Adapted from the AHA/ACSM Health/Fitness Facility Preparticipation Screening Questionnaire
Key: COPD = chronic obstructive pulmonary disease; GP = general practitioner

Once the individual has completed the questionnaire, they can be classified into one of three categories: *low risk* (or apparently healthy), *moderate risk* and *high risk* (see Table 11.1). This process is known as *risk stratification*.

The ACSM states that individuals who have two or more risk factors, men who are 45 or older and women who are 55 or older have a moderate risk factor. It is not recommended that individuals in this category be prescribed any vigorous exercise unless medical approval is given. Individuals in the high-risk category should not be allowed to exercise unless supervised by a qualified person.

NEED TO KNOW

If an individual has an HDL cholesterol reading under 1.6 mmol/l, subtract one risk factor from their total.

Health and safety issues

It is important for health and fitness instructors to be aware that they need to address many health and safety issues due to the emerging litigational environment that they work in and,

more importantly, for the safety of their clients. The main areas for concern are health and safety at work, equipment management, risk assessment, emergency first aid and potential accidents/incidents.

Health and safety at work

As in any environment, health and safety is an issue in any facility in which exercise is undertaken. A selection of the roles relevant to the health and fitness instructor is as follows:

1. Take responsible care for their own safety and that of others.
2. Cooperate with employers in matters of safety.
3. Do not interfere with or misuse anything provided for safety.

Larger health and fitness organizations should, by law, make a health and safety policy statement available to all staff and provide employees with relevant training. However, prior to working in any health and fitness environment the instructor must be familiar with several fundamental safety issues. It is in the interest of instructors to identify and familiarize themselves with the normal operating procedures and emergency operating procedures (EOPs) in the workplace to become aware of procedures that could help to minimize the occurrence of accident or injury.

Table 11.1	Risk factor stratification
Low (apparently healthy)	Younger individuals (men under 45 and women under 55) who are asymptomatic and have no more than one risk factor
Moderate	Older individuals (men 45 or older and women 55 or older) or those with two or more risk factors
High	Individuals with one or more sign/symptom of coronary heart disease or those with known cardiovascular, pulmonary or metabolic disease

Equipment management

The management of equipment during an exercise session is important with respect to overall safety. Equipment should not form an obstruction to the participants who are in the facility. For example, free weights should always be returned to their correct storage rack. It is also important to check equipment, such as pulleys and cables, for any wear and tear or malfunction prior to use. Instructors should also know how to operate any equipment and be able to locate manufacturers' manuals or guides. These guides should indicate the type and frequency of maintenance required.

Risk assessment

Any form of exercise or physical activity carries risks. Although these risks cannot be eradicated completely, they can be recognized, addressed and minimized. When planning an exercise session, it is advisable to complete and document a risk assessment. This acts as a written reminder for the instructor as well as providing evidence that preventive steps were taken, should an accident occur. Figure 11.3 provides a template that can be used to formulate and document a basic risk assessment.

Emergency situations

During an exercise session, the instructor may have to deal with an emergency situation. If this occurs, the instructor should follow the procedure below:

1. **Assess the situation.** Approach quickly but remain calm. Identify any risks to yourself, the casualties and bystanders.
2. **Make the area safe.** The conditions that caused the emergency may need to be made safe.
3. **Give emergency aid.** Assess the casualty and give first aid.
4. **Get help.** Send someone for help or telephone for assistance.
5. **Comfort the casualty.** Comfort and reassure the casualty until help arrives.

Figure 11.3	Example risk assessment form		
Potential risk	Method of minimizing risk	Action to be taken	Done
Recovery from shoulder injury	Limit range of motion and weight	Set pec dec range to start at limited range of motion	?
Trips due to free weights on floor in gym area	Ensure members return free weights to storage when finished	Signs put up around gym area to instruct members to return free weights to storage	?

First aid

Employers must provide adequate equipment and facilities to enable first aid to be carried out on sick or injured employees. Although they are not required by law to provide for injured clients, instructors trained in first aid should make every attempt to administer first aid should the situation arise.

Accident/incident report

In the event of an accident or incident during a gym session in which the instructor is in charge, an accident/incident report must be completed as a record of the event. The facility at which the instructor is working must provide the relevant form. The instructor may also have to deal with emergency procedures such as fires, security incidents or missing persons. In these cases, it is important to follow the facility's EOPs. Instructors therefore need to familiarize themselves with these procedures at each site at which they work.

If an instructor needs to contact the emergency services, they must give clear and accurate information as regard the following:

- Own name
- Nature of emergency
- Details of any casualty
- Time of emergency
- Facility details
- Contact number

Prior to the arrival of the emergency services, the instructor must deal with the emergency in the correct manner. Any requirement for emergency first aid must be given and any minor injuries can be dealt with accordingly, otherwise, the casualty must be made as comfortable as possible. All staff at the center must be informed about the arrival of the emergency services so that clear access can be prepared in advance. As a simple guideline, the following procedure should be adhered to during an emergency situation:

1. Inform the people involved about the correct emergency procedures.
2. Follow procedures in a calm but correct manner.
3. Maintain the safety of those involved at all times.
4. Clearly and accurately report any problems to a responsible colleague.
5. Make a detailed report of the incident afterward.

EXAMPLE QUESTIONS

11.1 The PAR-Q is a screening questionnaire used to identify conditions prior to encouraging exercise at what level?

a) a vigorous level

b) a high intensity

c) a light- to -moderate intensity

d) all levels

11.2 How long is the PAR-Q valid for?

a) no time limit

b) six weeks

c) six months

d) 12 months

11.3 True or false? The PAR-Q is a confidential document.

True

False

11.4 Which of the following is classed as a risk factor in relation to family history?

a) myocardial infarction or sudden death before age 45 in father, brother or son; before age 65 in mother, sister or daughter

b) myocardial infarction or sudden death before age 55 in father, brother or son; before age 65 in mother, sister or daughter

c) myocardial infarction or sudden death before age 55 in father, brother or son; before age 75 in mother, sister or daughter

d) myocardial infarction or sudden death before age 55 in father, brother or son; before age 60 in mother, sister or daughter

11.5 Which of the following is classed as a risk factor in relation to hypertension?

a) systolic pressure of 120 mmHg or above, or diastolic pressure of 80 mmHg or above

b) systolic pressure of 140 mmHg or above, or diastolic pressure of 80 mmHg or above

c) systolic pressure of 120 mmHg or above, or diastolic pressure of 90 mmHg or above

d) systolic pressure of 140 mmHg or above, or diastolic pressure of 90 mmHg or above

EXAMPLE QUESTIONS cont.

11.6 Which of the following is classed as a risk factor in relation to obesity?
   a) BMI of 15 kg/m^2 or above
   b) BMI of 20 kg/m^2 or above
   c) BMI of 25 kg/m^2 or above
   d) BMI of 30 kg/m^2 or above

11.7 Which of the following is classed as a risk factor in relation to dyslipidemia?
   a) total serum cholesterol of more than 3.2 mmol/l
   b) total serum cholesterol of more than 6.2 mmol/l
   c) total serum cholesterol of more than 5.2 mmol/l
   d) total serum cholesterol of more than 4.2 mmol/l

11.8 Which of the following is classed as a risk factor in relation to dyslipidemia?
   a) LDL more than 3.4 mmol/l, or HDL less than 1.03 mmol/l
   b) LDL more than 3.2 mmol/l, or HDL less than 1.03 mmol/l
   c) LDL more than 3.4 mmol/l, or HDL less than 1.23 mmol/l
   d) LDL more than 4.4 mmol/l, or HDL less than 1.03 mmol/l

11.9 With regard to risk stratification, the ACSM states that which group of people is at moderate risk?
   a) men 45 or older and women 55 or older or those with three or more risk factors
   b) men 45 or older and women 65 or older or those with two or more risk factors
   c) men 45 or older and women 55 or older or those with two or more risk factors
   d) men 50 or older and women 60 or older or those with two or more risk factors

11.10 Which of the following is classed as a risk factor in relation to impaired fasting glucose?
   a) 140 mg/dl or more
   b) 80 mg/dl or more
   c) 100 mg/dl or more
   d) 120 mg/dl or more

EXAMPLE QUESTIONS cont.

11.11 With regard to risk stratification, which group of people does the ACSM classify as low risk?
- **a)** men under 55 and women under 65 who are asymptomatic and have no more than one risk factor
- **b)** men under 45 years and women under 55 who are asymptomatic and have no more than two risk factors
- **c)** men under 45 years and women under 55 years who are asymptomatic and have no more than one risk factor
- **d)** men under 40 years and women under 55 years who are asymptomatic and have no more than one risk factor

11.12 True or false? A sedentary lifestyle is classed as a risk factor for coronary heart disease.
True
False

Further reading

American College of Sports Medicine (2006) *ACSM Guidelines to Exercise Testing and Prescription* (7th ed.), Lippincott, Williams & Wilkins

Baechle, R.T. (2000) *Essentials of Strength Training and Conditioning*, Human Kinetics

Howley, E.T. and Franks, B.D. (1997) *Health and Fitness Instructor's Handbook* (3rd ed.), Human Kinetics

Sewell, D., Watkins, P. and Griffin, M. (2005) *Sport and Exercise Science: An Introduction*, Hodder Arnold

NOTES

BEHAVIORAL CHANGE AND GOAL SETTING

12

OBJECTIVES

After completing this chapter, you will be able to

1 List and describe the stages of the Prochaska and DiClemente 'Stages of Change' model.

2 List and describe the cognitive and behavioral processes relating to the stages of change model.

3 Relate the cognitive and behavioral processes to the appropriate stage of change.

4 List various motivational factors relating to individuals initiating or maintaining an exercise program.

5 Explain how goal setting can be used in an exercise environment.

Instructing Exercise and Fitness Knowledge

Basic Anatomy and Physiology

- The importance of careful and thorough planning and preparation for sessions.

- How to identify and agree on objectives for the session based upon collected information.

- The goals of the designated programs that you are helping to deliver.

- The needs and potential of the participants, including reasons for and barriers to participation in the appropriate activity.

Instructing Physical Activity and Exercise Knowledge

Behavior Change

- Individual history and attitude to exercise:
  - Identifying and understanding the psychological benefits of exercise
  - Identifying the potential barriers to exercise participation
  - Principles of behavioral change: the Stages of Change model (Prochaska and DiClemente)
  - Determinants of behavior change and the cognitive and behavioral processes to progress through the stages of change
  - Motivational and exercise adherence strategies:
    - programming/prescription strategies
    - the principles of motivational interviewing

- • behavioral and outcome goal setting
- • social support
- • social reinforcement
- • attentional strategies
■ Intervention/motivational methods appropriate for each stage of behavior change:
  - •Understanding why people relapse and relapse prevention strategies

Introduction

This chapter deals with the common processes of behavioral change and also goal-setting strategies. Instructors should be able to identify and describe common processes of behavioral change, as well as describe general methods of goal setting within the health and fitness industry.

Later chapters in the book provide information about program design that, along with the content covered in this chapter, provides the instructor with the understanding and ability to design appropriate exercise programs for apparently healthy individuals, in line with current guidelines for exercise.

Exercise psychology

As well as the physiologic benefits of exercise, there are many psychological benefits that play an important part in helping individuals to take up and maintain a regular program of exercise. The psychological effects of exercise can be difficult to measure; however, it is claimed anecdotally that exercise can improve subjective feelings such as self-esteem, mood, self-image and confidence. It is also thought that exercise can help to reduce stress and anxiety by providing a distraction.

Even though there are possible physiologic explanations for these psychological effects, such as endorphins released after exercise having a positive effect on mood, psychological strategies about exercise are considered to play an important role in uptake and adherence to exercise. One of the main areas of focus from a psychological perspective is finding strategies to help individuals overcome barriers to exercise by making permanent changes to their lifestyle and behavior. These barriers include lack of funds, poor self-image, lack of enjoyment and, primarily, lack of available time. Instructors within the health and fitness industry might choose to identify which barriers to exercise are relevant to their particular client by simply asking direct questions. Once these barriers have been identified, the instructor can devise strategies to help overcome them. For example, if lack of time is an issue, the instructor could suggest walking more briskly whenever there is a need to walk, or getting off the bus one stop earlier if the client uses public transport. The instructor could also choose to use psychological strategies that have been successful following many years of research. One such strategy is the 'behavioral change model' discussed below.

Behavioral change

Much of the adult population does not engage in any form of regular exercise; therefore, starting an exercise program often requires a change in lifestyle and habits on the part of the individual. This is sometimes known as *behavioral change*. It can be challenging for both the individual and the instructor to overcome habits that have been in place for many years as research has suggested that behavioral change is a long-term process. However, models such as Prochaska and DiClemente's 'Stages of Change' model can help instructors to facilitate the process.

Stages of Change model (Prochaska and DiClemente)

This model proposes that there are a number of stages to any lifestyle change, such as stopping smoking or alcohol rehabilitation. Indeed, the research carried out by Prochaska and DiClemente used smoking cessation as the theme for the conception of the model; however, it can also be applied to exercise uptake.

As can be seen from Figure 12.1, there are several stages of change that will vary in duration depending on the individual. Table 12.1 describes the stages of change in more detail.

It is interesting to note that stages of change in relation to exercise uptake are cyclical in nature: in other words, an individual can go from one stage to the next and back again without ever moving any further on in the model. Approximately 15 percent of all individuals will experience relapse to the contemplation or precontemplation stage. Depending on which stage of the model the individual is at, it can be

Table 12.1	Description of the 'Stages of Change' (Prochaska and DiClemente)
Stage	**Description**
Precontemplation (I won't)	The individual does not intend to take any action in the short term (within about six months)
Contemplation (I might)	The individual intends to take action soon but is unsure about the change
Preparation (I will)	The individual has taken steps toward action and is planning to act, usually within one month
Action (I am)	The individual has taken action and changed his/her behavior in the short term
Maintenance (I have)	Behavioral change has lasted more than six months and the individual is committed to the change
Relapse	This can happen at any stage and many times over

Figure 12.1 The 'Stages of Change' model

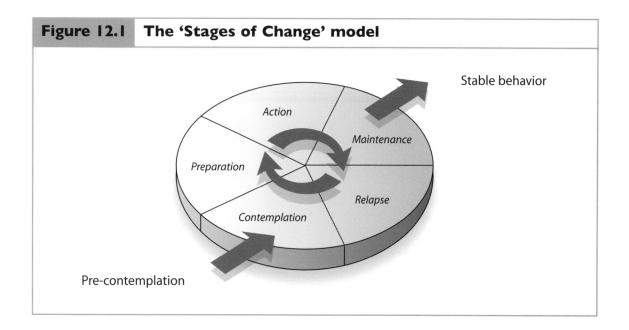

Stable behavior

Action

Maintenance

Preparation

Relapse

Contemplation

Pre-contemplation

important to provide help or support in order for the individual to progress through the stages. One of the strategies used for this purpose is that of *cognitive* and *behavioral processes.*

Cognitive and behavioral processes

The stage an individual is at can be ascertained by simple questioning during the screening and lifestyle sessions (see Chapter 11). Simply asking the individual which stage they think they are at is sometimes enough, or the answers they give to the instructor's questions can make it evident. Depending on the identified stage of change, the instructor can use strategies known as *cognitive* (experiential) and *behavioral processes* to help the individual, hopefully, to arrive at the maintenance stage.

Cognitive processes involve implementing changes to the way individuals think about lifestyle and are divided into five areas (see Table 12.2).

NEED TO KNOW

The 'Stages of Change' model is also known as the 'transtheoretical model.'

The cognitive processes outlined in Table 12.2 are usually adopted by individuals in the early stages of the 'Stages of Change' model, (precontemplation to preparation). Once the individual has moved to the action or maintenance stage, the cognitive processes are not as important as the individual has already thought about the exercise. At this stage the five *behavioral processes* listed in Table 12.3 can be more important.

Depending on which stage the individual is at, certain cognitive or behavioral processes are more likely to be successful in helping

Table 12.2	Cognitive processes
Cognitive processes	Description
Consciousness raising (increasing knowledge)	This relates to seeking new information and understanding, such as ascertaining the benefits of exercise and the risks associated with sedentary behavior. In terms of health and fitness, examples include visiting one's physician or talking to friends.
Dramatic relief (warning signs)	This relates to the feelings that can be experienced as a result of exercise or sedentary behavior, such as injury or pain, or tasks becoming more difficult as the individual ages.
Environmental reevaluation	This involves reflecting on how behavior can affect other people, such as being a role model and helping others, or sedentary behavior 'rubbing off' on a friend or partner.
Self-reevaluation	This can be related to reeducating the individual about beliefs related to exercise, such as exercise does not need to be painful to have good benefits, or exercise can prevent another heart attack.
Social liberation	This relates to helping oneself or others in similar situations and increasing awareness of exercise strategies.

them to move toward the next stage of change. Table 12.4 will guide the instructor to employ the most useful processes at various stages of change.

NEED TO KNOW

Many professional sports clubs employ psychologists to help implement motivational strategies.

Even though research is limited in the health and fitness environment in relation to exercise uptake, there is much anecdotal evidence to support the use of the processes. However, instructors should be aware of and focus on the move from the contemplation stage to the action stage as this is often reported to be the most difficult transition. Instructors should also be aware that many individuals will cite barriers that prevent them from exercising, such as lack of funds, lack of transport, no peer support and self-consciousness, among others. Therefore, it is the role of the instructor to devise strategies and suggest ways for the individual to overcome these potential barriers.

The psychological strategies discussed in this chapter have been shown to influence exercise adherence and, as such, positively impact on the benefits of a healthy lifestyle. As these psychological strategies extend beyond the scope of this book, instructors and individuals are encouraged to increase their knowledge of

Behavioral processes	Description
Table 12.3	**Behavioral processes**
Self-liberation (understanding the benefits)	This relates to experiencing the benefits of committing to exercise by taking responsibility, which can inspire confidence and self-belief. At this stage the instructor and the individual should make firm resolutions.
Helping relationships	This relates to providing and accepting support for the individual and encouraging empowerment. Buddy systems or personal trainers can be used here. Remind the individual why exercise can be good.
Reinforcement management (rewards)	This involves providing rewards such as T-shirts, badges and certificates for meeting goals and targets and punishment or forfeits for not.
Counterconditioning (alternatives)	This involves trying to focus on the positive changes of exercise choices replacing sedentary choices, such as using stairs instead of elevators or walking the dog instead of watching TV.
Stimulus control	This involves trying to remove options for sedentary behavior, such as hiding the TV remote control, switching on the radio as opposed to the TV and keeping exercise clothes prominent.

this particular area as part of self-development and progression. There are many sources available to the instructor (or individual) such as books, websites and courses that relate specifically to the health and fitness industry, in particular to areas such as exercise adherence, performance enhancement, team building, lifestyle management and injury rehabilitation.

TASK

List the 'stages of change' and explain how various cognitive and behavioral strategies can help individuals to move through the stages.

Motivation

The word 'motivate' is derived from the Latin for 'move' and can be defined as 'the internal mechanisms and external stimuli that arouse and direct our behavior.' In other words, motivation is what prompts a person to act. This can include the motivation to make lifestyle changes in order to affect weight loss or increase cardiovascular fitness, which relates directly to the cognitive and behavioral processes discussed previously.

In relation to exercise, individuals might have more than one motive to start or maintain an exercise program, and their motivation could change over a period of time. Many

Table 12.4	Processes most likely to aid movement toward the next 'stage of change'		
Contemplation	Preparation	Action	Maintenance
Consciousness raising: statistics on obesity, information about how exercise can reduce obesity, etc.	Self-reevaluation: small lifestyle changes can have benefits, etc.	Self-liberation: congratulations, you did it and it feels good!	Reinforcement management: well done, you've won a T-shirt for achieving your first goal
Dramatic relief: sedentary behavior makes you feel lethargic, but exercise makes you feel good, etc.			Helping relationships: train with a partner – this really helps
Environmental reevaluation: friends might want to join you, etc.			Counterconditioning: we have an agreement at work not to use the stairs, etc.
			Stimulus control: my partner only allows the remote after exercise, etc.

factors can affect motivational preference, so instructors must be aware that they need to regularly address this with the individual. Table 12.5 outlines some of the commonly cited motives for individuals who are either just starting an exercise program or maintaining an exercise program.

Types of motivation

Various motivational factors can influence training in different ways. Athletes may be highly motivated for competition reasons, whereas a beginner to exercise may be motivated by factors such as weight loss. These

Table 12.5	Common motives for starting/maintaining an exercise program
Starting	Maintaining
Health	Enjoyment
Appearance	Role model's influence
Guidance	Variation of activities
Challenge	Social
Submission	Self-esteem
Compulsion	Helping others
Fitness	

motivational factors may come from external sources such as a coach or a partner or from internal factors such as the individual themselves. These types of motivation are commonly referred to as *extrinsic* and *intrinsic* motivation.

Extrinsic motivation

This term is used when individuals are motivated to exercise by external rewards such as certificates, T-shirts, medals and trophies. Many people are motivated extrinsically, so it is prudent to ascertain which extrinsic motivational factors an individual responds best to. However, external rewards can be motivational providing they are not the only reason for taking part in exercise. For adherence reasons, it is also important to make sure that individuals are not overreliant on external rewards but focus on internal motivational factors as well.

Intrinsic motivation

This term is used when individuals are motivated to exercise by factors such as enjoyment, fun or self-satisfaction. This type of motivation can be linked to outcome goals (see page 188): for example when an individual achieves a certain exercise goal it could lead to a positive feeling of self-achievement. It might be beneficial to try and identify the type of motivational strategy that might suit the individual during the initial consultation. This can be done by questioning the individual about past exercise history and the success or failure of that exercise history. If a motivational preference cannot be established, try employing motivational techniques, such as those listed below, to assess if they have a positive or negative effect.

Common motivational techniques

Below are some common motivational techniques to try with clients:

1. To start with, set short-term goals that are easily achievable.
2. Encourage the individual to find a training partner (use a buddy system).
3. Keep an exercise diary for visual effect.
4. If weight loss is a goal, use pictures of the individual when he or she was slimmer as an incentive to get back to that size.
5. Keep a reminder in a prominent place (on the individual's desk or fridge door) of the reasons why the individual wants to achieve their specific goals: for example wanting to increase cardiovascular fitness to run in a charity fun run in six months' time.
6. Introduce the individual to other activities and social events within the exercise facility.
7. Encourage the individual to keep their exercise kit in a prominent place.

TASK

Briefly define the term 'motivation' and list the various extrinsic and intrinsic motivational techniques that are commonly used in the health and fitness industry.

Goal setting

Goal setting is a simple, yet often misused motivational technique that can provide some structure for an exercise program. Goals are usually set in order to accomplish a specific task in a specific period of time, such as losing a certain amount of weight for a wedding or being able to run a half-marathon in six months' time. Goal setting can provide a plan of action to help the individual to focus and direct their activities. Regardless of the ability level, fitness status, experience or motivation of the individual, goal setting can be a valuable tool not just for the instructor but for the individual as well.

Generally speaking, in relation to exercise there are two categories of goal setting: *process goals* and *outcome goals*. Process goals are goals where the skill is broken down into manageable units for the subject to focus on. Often form and technique can be classed as process goals as they are task-related rather than results-related. Outcome goals are concerned only with the ultimate outcome, for example success or failure, winning or losing. In other words, outcome goals are results-related as opposed to task-related. Focus on outcome goals can often affect attention to process goals, which can result in a detrimental effect on the outcome.

Therefore, instructors and individuals should try to focus on process goals as well as outcome goals in the initial stages of an exercise program. Typical process and outcome goals are outlined in Table 12.6.

The SMARTER principle

Goals in relation to exercise can be set for the short-, medium- and long-term. If only long-term goals were set, the individual might lose interest and exercise adherence could be affected, whereas achievement of short-term goals could act as a motivational tool for the individual. When agreeing goals with the individual, whether short-, medium- or long-term, the acronym *SMART* or *SMARTER* is a useful guide and includes several common characteristics that are often associated with effective goal setting (see Table 12.7).

Table 12.6 Common process and outcome goals	
Process goals	Outcome goals
• Be able to do free-weight exercises • Be able to run or jog without heart pounding • Establish a routine • Enjoy the exercise • Exercise on your own	• Reduce body fat percentage • Decrease blood pressure • Increase VO_{2max} • Complete a marathon • Reduce a dress size

Table 12.7   Examples of SMARTER goals

S	Goals must be **Specific**.	If an individual wants to follow a weight-loss program, be specific about the amount of weight loss that is set as the target. For instance, 0.5 kg per week could be a specific target.
M	Training targets should be **Measurable**.	In the example above, 0.5 kg per week is a measurable amount, as opposed to 'lose a little weight each week.'
A	Goals should be **Adjustable**.	If an individual finds the target too easy or too hard, the instructor must adapt the program to suit. In other words, the program must be adjustable.
R	Goals must be **Realistic**.	Set targets that are achievable: 0.5 kg weight loss per week is an achievable target for most people, whereas a target of over 3 kg per week might not be achievable by all people.
T	Training targets should be **Time-based**.	For example, 0.5 kg weight loss per week can be a short-term target that can lead to an overall loss of about 26 kg a year, which is a long-term goal.
E	Goals should be challenging and **Exciting**.	The chances of adherence to the program are much greater if the program is exciting in some way.
R	Goals should be **Recorded**.	Make sure that the individual keeps a record of exercise activity as this provides a visual stimulus for the individual and prevents any confusion over a longer term.

EXAMPLE QUESTIONS

12.1 The 'Stages of Change' model follows what type of pattern?
  a) rhythmical
  b) cyclical
  c) exponential
  d) linear

12.2 Approximately what percentage of all individuals will experience relapse back to the contemplation or precontemplation stage?
  a) 5 percent
  b) 10 percent
  c) 15 percent
  d) 20 percent

12.3 True or false? Cognitive processes are usually adopted by individuals in the early stages of the 'Stages of Change' model, from not thinking about exercise to taking up exercise.
  True
  False

12.4 True or false? Behavioral processes are usually adopted by individuals in the later stages of the 'Stages of Change' model.
  True
  False

12.5 What is the following a definition of: 'the internal mechanisms and external stimuli that arouse and direct our behavior.'?
  a) cognitive process
  b) behavioral process
  c) goal setting
  d) motivation

EXAMPLE QUESTIONS cont.

12.6 Which term is used to describe an individual being motivated to exercise by factors such as enjoyment, fun or self-satisfaction?

a) intrinsic motivation

b) extrinsic motivation

c) external motivation

d) behavioral motivation

12.7 When a skill is broken down into manageable units that the subject can focus on, it is known as what type of goal?

a) SMART

b) outcome

c) process

d) realistic

12.8 Goals that are concerned only with the ultimate outcome, for example success or failure, winning or losing, are known as what type of goal?

a) SMART

b) outcome

c) process

d) realistic

12.9 In the acronym SMARTER, what does the first R stand for?

a) resistance

b) recordable

c) realistic

d) ready

12.10 In the acronym SMARTER, what does the M stand for?

a) machines

b) measurable

c) motivate

d) mentor

EXAMPLE QUESTIONS cont.

12.11 In the acronym SMARTER, what does the S stand for?

a) service

b) specific

c) supervise

d) set

12.12 In the acronym SMARTER, what does the A stand for?

a) adjustable

b) amount

c) achievable

d) action

Further reading

American College of Sports Medicine (2006) *ACSM Guidelines to Exercise Testing and Prescription* (7th ed), Lippincott, Williams & Wilkins

Atkinson, R. (1996) *Introduction to Psychology*, Harcourt Brace Jovanovich College Publishers

Bull, S.J. (1996) *Sport Psychology: A Self-help Guide*, Crowood

Cox, R.H. (1994) *Sport Psychology Concepts and Applications*, Brown & Benchmark

Horn, T. (1996) *Advances in Sport Psychology*, Human Kinetics

Howley, E.T. and Franks, B.D. (1997) *Health Fitness Instructor's Handbook* (3rd ed.), Human Kinetics

Jackson, S.A. and Csikszentmihalyi, M. (1999) *Flow in Sports*, Human Kinetics

Kremer, J.M. and Scully, D.M. (1994) *Psychology in Sport*, Taylor & Francis

Murphy, S.M. (1995) *Sport Psychology Interventions*, Human Kinetics

Orlick, T. (1998) *Embracing Your Potential*, Human Kinetics

Williams, J.M. (1998) *Applied Sport Psychology: Personal growth to peak performance* (3rd ed.), Mayfield

NOTES

COMPONENTS AND INDUCTION OF AN EXERCISE SESSION

OBJECTIVES

After completing this chapter, you will be able to

1 Explain the term 'induction' in relation to exercise sessions.

2 Describe the process of warm-up, cardio, cool-down and resistance and flexibility inductions for beginners to exercise.

3 List the common guidelines relating to the use of cardiovascular equipment.

4 List and describe the components of an exercise session.

5 List and describe each of the 'cardio training zones.'

6 Briefly describe the terms 'interval' and 'fartlek' in relation to cardio training.

7 Describe the term 'resistance exercise continuum.'

8 Explain the term 'periodization' and list its components.

Instructing Exercise and Fitness Knowledge

Basic Anatomy and Physiology

- The application of the principles and variables of fitness to the components of fitness.
- How to apply the principles and variables of fitness to a range of activities that will achieve various health benefits and the required fitness development.
- The importance of careful and thorough planning and preparation for sessions.
- The goals of the designated programs that you are helping to deliver.
- How to apply the principles and variables of fitness to a range of activities that will achieve various health benefits and the required fitness development.
- The program/session card and how to record plans on it.

Instructing Physical Activity and Exercise Knowledge

Components of fitness

- Heart-rate training zones

- Components of fitness:
  - Aerobic capacity
  - Muscular strength
  - Muscular resistance
  - Flexibility
- Rep ranges for strength, power, endurance and hypertrophy
- American College of Sports Medicine guidelines for developing each component of fitness
- Continuum between muscular strength and muscular endurance
- Interval and fartlek training – principles and practice
- Principles of periodization
  - Macro-, meso- and microcycles
  - Volume vs intensity through the cycles
- Importance of rest and signs and symptoms of overtraining

Introduction

This chapter deals with the components of an exercise session. Instructors should be able to identify the components of an exercise session and list the guidelines associated with them.

This chapter, along with others in the book, provides information regarding the practical application of theoretical knowledge. This will allow the instructor to design appropriate exercise programs for apparently healthy individuals, in line with current guidelines for exercise.

Components of an exercise session

A typical exercise session forming part of an overall exercise program would normally include the following components, as recommended by the American College of Sports Medicine (ACSM):

1. Warm-up
2. Conditioning phase (including cardio, resistance and flexibility training)
3. Cool-down.

Warm-up

Prior to the exercise session, it is essential that the body (and in particular the connective tissues) is fully warmed in order to reduce the potential for injury. Research has shown that perhaps the main factor in muscular injury prevention is muscle temperature: muscle is more elastic when warm and therefore less susceptible to injury.

The entire warm-up should take about 5–10 minutes and should facilitate the transition from rest to the level of exercise required in the main session. The intensity of the warm-up should increase gradually in order to avoid the onset of oxygen debt and can be performed using cardiovascular equipment, such as a treadmill, rower, or cycle or step machine or, if no equipment is available, through brisk walking or slow jogging. There is very little difference in the benefits of each method as they are all capable of stressing the cardiorespiratory system.

The warm-up should aim to achieve a change in a number of physiologic responses, in order that the body can work safely and effectively. Typical benefits of a warm-up are

1. An increase in body temperature, specifically core muscle temperature
2. An increase in the elasticity of muscular tissues
3. A decreased risk of soft-tissue injury
4. Activation of the neuromuscular system
5. An increase in mental alertness
6. Release of synovial fluid.

Conditioning phase

According to the ACSM, the conditioning phase of an exercise session should include one or more of the following types of training: cardiovascular, resistance and flexibility. For a comprehensive session, all areas are recommended.

Cardiovascular training

The cardiovascular session should follow on from the warm-up and can involve the same type of cardiovascular equipment. At the end of the warm-up the heart rate should be at the level required for the cardiovascular session, depending on the goal of the individual. Guidelines for the recommended heart-rate levels and duration and frequency of exercise can be taken from the ACSM guidelines.

Benefits of cardiovascular training

The main benefits of cardiovascular training, dependent on the intensity, frequency and duration of the exercise, are

1. Weight (fat) loss due to an increase in fat metabolism
2. Increased glycogen stores
3. Increased aerobic and anaerobic enzymes
4. Increase in the number and size of mitochondria
5. Increased number of capillaries
6. Increased myoglobin levels
7. Increased recruitment of muscle fibers
8. Increased self-confidence and self-esteem.

NEED TO KNOW

For an average individual it is recommended that energy expenditure per day from exercise should be between 300 and 400 kcal.

Cardio training zones

When prescribing cardiovascular exercise, the intensity (how hard the individual should exercise) should be carefully considered. Before agreeing on the level of the exercise with an individual, it is useful to understand the benefits of exercising at different levels of intensity, otherwise known as *cardio training zones* (see Figure 13.1). In basic terms, each specific training zone is related to a heart-rate range in which certain benefits might be expected. The zones are not exact, but they are useful as a guide to cardiovascular training as the benefits relating to each zone are reasonably accurate.

Figure 13.1	**Cardio training zones**

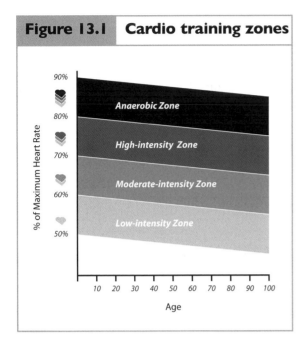

Training zones are based on a percentage window (60–70 percent, for example) of maximum heart rate (MHR). Within each training zone, subtle physiologic effects take place in relation to the heart rate.

Low-intensity zone: 50–60 percent MHR

This training zone is mainly suitable for deconditioned individuals, or individuals who cannot maintain a normal conversation within the heart-rate levels specific to this zone. Regular exercise in this zone will lead to slight improvements in cardiovascular function, depending on the frequency and duration of the exercise undertaken.

Exercise sessions within this zone might only last for a few minutes, so the minimum goal of 20 minutes of cardiovascular exercise, as recommended by the ACSM, should become a target for the client to achieve comfortably before progressing to higher intensity levels such as those in the weight-management zone.

Moderate-intensity zone: 60–70 percent MHR

Training within this zone develops endurance and aerobic capacity, again depending on the frequency and duration of the exercise undertaken. Exercising in this zone also burns fat at a higher rate than the previous zone, which is associated with weight loss. There should also be an overall improvement in the health status and cardiorespiratory function of the individual.

At this level of intensity, most individuals will be aware of an increase in heart rate but should be able to carry out a normal conversation. The weight-management zone should be achievable for most beginners to exercise and should be sufficient to bring about overload and hence adaptation to the demands of the exercise. From an exercise adherence perspective, this zone can be beneficial to beginners in that they should feel reasonably comfortable with the level of intensity but should also experience the benefits of adaptation. As the benefits of cardiovascular exercise are affected by frequency, duration and intensity, it is suggested that duration should follow the ACSM guidelines of 20–60 minutes, at a frequency of three to five days per week. In terms of intensity, a greater amount of energy will be expended at 70 percent of MHR compared with that expended at 60 percent for the same amount of time; this will affect the overall amount of fat used as fuel for the exercise.

High-intensity zone: 70–80 percent MHR

This zone is sometimes referred to as the 'fitness' zone. The ability of the body to transport oxygen to and carbon dioxide away from the working muscles can be developed and improved by training in this zone. At this level of intensity breathing rate is increased, so this level is more appropriate for individuals who are used to exercising on a regular basis. Some individuals will still be able to carry out a conversation at this level, but others might find it difficult to do so while still maintaining regular breathing.

Anaerobic zone: 80–90 percent MHR

Training in this zone can help to develop the lactic acid system (see Chapter 6). In this zone the individual's anaerobic threshold is normally reached. The amount of fat used (in percentage terms) as the main source of energy in this zone is greatly reduced as glycogen stored in the muscle is the predominant source of fuel. One of the by-products of using glycogen as a fuel is lactic acid. The body can normally remove and deal with low levels of lactic acid, but as levels of lactic acid start to increase the body reaches a point at which it can no longer remove the lactic acid from the working muscles quickly enough. This happens at a heart rate, and hence intensity, that is specific to each individual and is usually accompanied by a rapid rise in heart rate and a slowing of intensity. This point is known as the *onset of blood lactate* or *OBLA*. The correct type of training can increase the body's ability to remove lactic acid for a longer period of time, thus delaying the OBLA. Due to the high-intensity levels associated with this zone, it is mainly suitable for athletes or those individuals who have a considerable base of fitness. It is important to note that at higher intensity levels such as these, the risk of orthopedic injuries and cardiac complications is increased.

Duration of cardiovascular training

Regardless of the training zone being used, the guidelines for cardiovascular endurance as stated by the ACSM suggest a duration of 20–60 minutes continuous or intermittent exercise (intermittent meaning an accumulation of 10-minute bouts of exercise throughout the day). A distinction should be made between this definition and intermittent types of cardiovascular training that are sometimes used by individuals as a training method. Two common types of intermittent cardiovascular training are *fartlek* and *interval training*.

Fartlek

The term fartlek loosely translates as 'speed play' and involves alternating the intensity level throughout the duration of the cardiovascular session. This kind of training appears to be random in relation to recovery periods and intensity levels.

Interval training

Interval training is a more systematic form of training that uses precise work:recovery ratios. For example, an individual will maintain a constant speed for a certain period of time at an aerobic level and then increase the intensity to an anaerobic level for a short period of time. The intensity will then be reduced to a lower level than at the start to allow the individual to recover. The process then begins again.

There is a complex interaction between the exact levels of aerobic and anaerobic intensity and the period of recovery, and a number of sessions are normally required in order to fine-tune this. Figure 13.2 provides an example of one cycle in an interval training session and can be explained as follows:

Figure 13.2 — Example of an interval training session

- **A–B:** This is the individual's normal level of aerobic intensity.
- **B–C:** The intensity is gradually increased to an anaerobic level.
- **C–D:** The anaerobic level is maintained for a short period of time.
- **D–E:** The level is quickly lowered in order to recover.
- **E–F:** The intensity is increased to the starting level.
- **F:** The process repeats itself.

Because of the high-intensity levels associated with interval and fartlek training, a higher degree of physical stress is placed on the structures of the body, especially at the joints. It is advisable for an individual to have an adequate cardiovascular base of fitness before undertaking this type of exercise. As all of the energy systems in the body are used during this type of training (see Chapter 6), careful planning is needed to target the systems so that the individual can achieve his or her goals. The following points should be considered:

1. The current fitness level of the individual.
2. The fitness goals of the individual.

3. The energy systems applicable to the goals identified.
4. The duration and intensity of the build-up to the required level.
5. The duration and intensity of recovery periods.
6. The duration and intensity of the normal work periods.
7. The number of repetitions of each cycle (overall duration).

NEED TO KNOW

Although constant rhythmic exercise is preferred by the ACSM, sports such as tennis and netball can be used in the cardiovascular conditioning phase.

Cool-down following a cardiovascular workout

The *cool-down,* is sometimes referred to as a *warm-down* and these two terms can be used interchangeably. Due to the increased heart rate of the cardiovascular part of the session, individuals need to take time to gradually reduce the heart rate and blood pressure to near resting levels. This is known as the cool-down.

The ACSM recommends a period of approximately five to 10 minutes for this part of the exercise session. Individuals can use the same type of cardiovascular equipment used in the warm-up and cardiovascular endurance sessions to achieve this but at a level that gradually reduces in intensity. In general terms, the cool-down should help to

1. Disperse lactic acid
2. Prevent blood pooling
3. Return the body systems to normal levels
4. Assist in maintaining venous return

5. Reduce the potential for hypotension and dizziness
6. Help to dissipate body heat.

NEED TO KNOW

As a general guide, the intensity levels of the exercise should be reduced gradually throughout the cool-down until the heart rate is below 100 bpm.

Cool-down guidelines

* Reduce the level of intensity gradually
* Elicit feedback from participants on the level of intensity
* Be in a position to observe all participants
* Stretches can be included on the move if the client is balanced.

Resistance training

Resistance training can be performed using different forms of exercise, such as resistance machines, free weights and body-weight exercises. Depending on the facility, a large range of resistance machines and free weights will be available. Prior to working with clients at a new facility, instructors should familiarize themselves with the machines when working at a new facility. The resistance training part of the session should start with a warm-up and finish with a cool-down.

Benefits of resistance training

Many benefits are associated with resistance training, depending on the intensity of the resistance, the number of sets and repetitions performed, the rest periods and many other variables. Common benefits include

1. Reduced risk of osteoporosis
2. Increase in muscle mass
3. Increase in bone mass
4. Increase in glucose tolerance
5. Increased joint integrity
6. Reduced back pain
7. Improved posture
8. Reduction of hypertension
9. Reduced risk of diabetes
10. Increased strength of connective tissue.

Warm-up for resistance training

It is not advisable to perform any muscular contractions against a resistance until the muscle or muscle groups have been prepared. This can be done by performing a number of contractions using a lighter weight than prescribed for each resistance exercise in the program.

Main activity

Prior to designing an exercise program that includes resistance training, it is necessary to establish the number of repetitions to be performed during the training session. This can be done either during the individual's induction or during the first training session. For example, if an individual decides to perform 10 repetitions, he or she needs to find a weight that they can lift successfully 10 times but fail on the 11th repetition. If the individual can perform more than 10 repetitions easily, the weight should be increased; if the individual cannot perform 10 repetitions, the weight should be decreased. This is a trial and error method that becomes easier to administer as the instructor gains experience.

The resistance exercise continuum

Common goals for a resistance training program include muscular strength, endurance,

Figure 13.3 The resistance exercise continuum

*Adapted from Baechle and Earle (2000)
Increasing darkness of color and increasing font size correspond to increased adaptation for the relevant goal at the repetition maximum.

hypertrophy and power. Training programs are normally devised in relation to the specific goal but can differ depending on the level of knowledge and experience of the individual. Although there is no such thing as an optimum program for muscular strength, endurance, hypertrophy or power gains due to the many variables that can affect the nature of a resistance training program, there is a general and commonly used guide that shows the intensity required to elicit specific gains. This is known as the *resistance exercise continuum* (see Figure 13.3).

In simple terms, to elicit strength gains it is logical to train with heavy loads, so the number of repetitions performed will be low. If, on the other hand, muscular endurance is the goal, it is logical to train with lighter loads and therefore perform a higher number of repetitions.

Depending on the outcome goal (strength, endurance, power or hypertrophy), a certain range of repetitions is recommended to elicit the appropriate adaptation, as can be seen in Figure 13.3. This range is not exact, and there is a certain degree of overlap due to the many variables that can affect adaptation to the specific training. The amount of weight (intensity) to be used can be based on a percentage of the individual's 1 repetition max (see pages 224–25).

NEED TO KNOW

Research has found little difference, in terms of adaptation, between single-set and multiple-set resistance training programs.

Free weights versus resistance machines

One of the current anecdotal debates within the health and fitness industry is whether to advocate free-weight exercises, resistance-machine exercises or both. Resistance machines vary greatly between manufacturers with respect to ergonomic design, range of adjustment and planes of movement, so it is impossible to advocate one method of resistance training over another. The advantages and disadvantages of both resistance machines and free weights must be taken into account on an individual basis (see Table 13.1). It is the instructor's responsibility to advise individuals of the benefits of both methods of resistance training and to take into account the individual's preference before designing an exercise program.

Table 13.1	Advantages and disadvantages of different types of resistance training	
	Advantages	Disadvantages
Free weights	• Many exercises can be performed with limited equipment. • Uses synergists and stabilizers in a functional isotonic way. • Full range of motion is available. • Less expensive compared with machines. • Relatively portable.	• More instruction required for safety and correct technique. • Often require a training partner for safety purposes. • Do not always appeal to a broad range of users.
Resistance machines	• Relatively easy to learn and therefore to instruct. • The weight selected does not need to be calculated. • The weight setting can be changed easily.	• The plane of motion is set by the machine, which is not functional. • Can sometimes limit range of motion. • Seated positions do not replicate most functional movements. • Seat supports negate the use of core stabilizers. • Lack of synergist and stabilizer use. • Relatively expensive compared with free weights.

Structure of the resistance training session

Regardless of whether resistance machines, free weights or both are incorporated into a training program, within each training session the larger muscle groups should be exercised before the smaller muscle groups. This is to prevent the smaller muscle groups from becoming fatigued and affecting the exercises in which they assist the larger muscle groups. For example, if the tricep muscles were exercised to fatigue before the bench press was performed, the individual would achieve a lower than normal weight, as the tricep muscles assist the pectorals in this exercise.

Cool-down following resistance training

The requirements of a cool-down following resistance training are similar to those following cardiovascular training (see pages 199–200). At the end of each exercise, the individual should perform several repetitions of the same exercise using a lighter weight than that used in the main activity.

Flexibility training

Flexibility is the range of possible movement in a joint. Flexibility exercises can be performed prior to the main cardio session after the warm-up or at the end of the cool-down, depending on preference. Recent ACSM guidelines for stretching state that static stretching reduces strength and should therefore only be done at the end of a workout. They should be performed a specific number of times per week at a certain intensity: two to four reps of 15–30 seconds.

The stretching exercises included within each exercise session should be related to the specific muscle groups that were used during the session.

Many stretches are in use throughout the health and fitness industry, and the type of stretch employed can depend on several factors, including the preference of the instructor who is designing the exercise program. However, certain stretches can place unnecessary strain on particular joints. These stretches are known as *contraindicated* stretches and should be avoided. Table 13.2 describes some typical stretches used in the health and fitness industry. For the purpose of this book, however, the focus will be upon stretches that are not considered to be contraindicated.

As with the other components of health-related physical fitness, it is essential that the instructor performs the correct technique when demonstrating any stretches in order for the client to copy.

TASK

List the components of an exercise session and briefly outline the ACSM recommendations relating to each component.

Periodization

The term 'periodization' is used in both sport and health and fitness. It relates to program design and the process of manipulation of a program of exercise at regular intervals, known as cycles. Although periodization is used predominantly by athletes in order to organize their training programs so that they 'peak' at competition times, it is also used in the health and fitness industry as a goal-setting tool: the regular manipulation of an exercise program is thought to elicit optimal gains in one or more of the components of fitness.

Table 13.2 Typical stretches

Muscles stretched	Key points	Demonstration
• Pectoralis major • Anterior deltoid	1. Stand with your feet hip-width apart. 2. Clasp your hands behind your back. 3. Straighten your arms. 4. Raise your arms until you feel tension. 5. Maintain neutral spine.	
• Trapezius • Latissimus dorsi • Posterior deltoid • Bicep brachii	1. Stand with your feet hip-width apart. 2. Clasp your hands in front of you. 3. Straighten your arms away from your body. 4. Separate the scapula by pushing your shoulders forward.	

Table 13.2	Typical stretches cont.	
Muscles stretched	Key points	Demonstration
• Triceps	1. Stand with your feet hip-width apart. 2. Raise one elbow above your head. 3. Reach toward the opposite scapula. 4. Increase the stretch by pushing your elbow with the opposite hand.	
• Hip flexors	1. Adopt the lunge position. 2. Lower the hips forward and down. 3. Keep your body upright. 4. Keep your front foot flat.	

Table 13.2	Typical stretches cont.	
Muscles stretched	**Key points**	**Demonstration**
• Quadriceps	1. Clasp the front of your foot. 2. Take your heel toward your bottom. 3. Keep your knees almost together. 4. Maintain neutral spine.	
• Hamstrings	1. Sit on the floor with neutral spine. 2. Place the heel of one foot on the inside of the opposite knee. 3. Lean forward from the waist. 4. Maintain neutral spine.	

Table 13.2 Typical stretches cont.

Muscles stretched	Key points	Demonstration
• Hip adductors	1. Sit on the floor with your legs wide apart. 2. Lean to one side, facing forward. 3. Bend the knee of the side to which you are leaning. 4. Keep the opposite leg straight.	
• Hip abductors	1. Sit on the floor with one leg out straight in front of you. 2. Cross the opposite leg over the straight leg. 3. Sit upright and hug your knee to your chest.	

In order to achieve this, it is common to monitor ongoing performance so that the program can be adjusted accordingly depending on the nature of the results. The program can be organized into intervals known as cycles. Each type of cycle has a different time allocation:

- **Microcycle:** This is the shortest period of training within an exercise program and normally refers to the number of training sessions in a seven-day period (that is short-term planning). Obviously, any goals within such a short period of time need to be achievable in relation to the individual.
- **Mesocycle:** This is a repeating series of microcycles over a period of several weeks (that is medium-term planning). The goals in a mesocycle should be achievable yet flexible as they can be manipulated following analysis of the microcycles within it.
- **Macrocycle:** This is a series of mesocycles, normally over a period of a few months to several years (that is long-term planning). Information gathered from microcycles and mesocycles can be used to confirm or readjust the long-term goals of the macrocycle.

Each microcycle contributes to the goals of the mesocycles, which in turn will contribute to the goals of the overall macrocycle. It is important that the instructor constantly revises the goals of each cycle due to the constant interaction of one cycle on another. Planning a program of exercise using periodized cycles can be useful as it can give individual short-, medium- and long-term goals (see Chapter 12). This has been shown to have a positive effect on adherence to exercise, not only for beginners but for regular exercisers as well. When designing an exercise program, it is recommended that it is recorded simply and

accurately so that the individual can use it as a reference during exercise sessions.

Recording exercise programs

There are many ways of recording exercise programs, but for a session within a microcycle it is common to use a session card (see Figure 13.4) that provides information relating to one session only. A typical session card contains all the information relevant to the individual performing the exercise, as well as information regarding the specific exercise plan. Be aware that information contained on a session card can be confidential, so it must be treated as such.

Induction sessions

The term *induction* is used to describe the process of the instructor explaining to the client the details and requirements of the exercise session in relation to their specific program, and showing them how the exercise session will be carried out in the environment they are going to use. For example, inductions that take place in a gym aim to familiarize the client with the operation of the equipment and the performance of the exercises in relation to the session. Therefore, as well as explaining how to operate any equipment, the induction should take the client through each component of the exercise session in turn (warm-up, cardio, cool-down, resistance and flexibility) to make sure they understand and practice each component. This will also give the instructor the opportunity to identify client training intensities in relation to cardiovascular and resistance equipment settings.

Figure 13.4	Example session plan template

SESSION PLAN: **Number:** **Page:**

Instructor name: **Client name:** **Ability level:**

Objectives:

Duration (reps, seconds, circuits etc.)	Exercises (name muscles used and draw diagrams where needed)	Equipment	Sets	Intensity (speed, rpm, weight, level)	Alternative and progression (and coaching points)

First aid point: **Tel:**

Resources: **Music:**

Client induction sessions are normally carried out following a successful client screening session (see Chapter 11) in which it was agreed that the client could begin a program of exercise. There are no specific guidelines relating to client induction procedures, which is one of the reasons why all health and fitness facilities tend to have their own methods for client induction. However, regardless of the method used for induction sessions, common guidelines can be applied. These guidelines relate to a client induction for the cardiovascular, resistance and flexibility components of the session to be performed.

Warm-up, cardio and cool-down induction

The facility in which the instructor is working will determine the type of cardiovascular machines available. When working at a new facility, instructors are advised to familiarize themselves with the machines prior to inducting individuals.

Before individuals begin a program of exercise, they need to be given an induction relating to their specific exercise program, starting with the first session. Following an explanation of the controls of the cardiovascular machines, it is usual for the instructor to take the individual through the training session in order to establish cardiovascular intensity levels for the warm-up, main activity and cool-down. There are many methods of inducting individuals on cardiovascular machines depending on the individual instructor's preference. However, in order to be consistent in the delivery, it is advisable to use a logical approach such as the acronym IDEA, which can be used regardless of the cardiovascular machine being used:

I Introduce the exercise
D Demonstrate the correct technique
E Explain the exercise using minimal coaching points
A Activity: observe the client doing the activity on the machine

It is important that instructors use correct technique when demonstrating so that the individual does not copy 'bad' technique. As the visual demonstration will provide a great deal of information for the individual, the verbal information that supplements this can be kept to a minimum. When the individual is using the machine, the instructor should maintain a dialogue in order to give them relevant information on performance and technique. The instructor should then aim to identify the suitable training intensity.

Even though a vast range of cardiovascular training equipment is available, there are many common guidelines that can be employed when using the equipment (see Table 13.3).

The treadmill can be used for both walking and running but is associated with greater impact on the joints than other cardiovascular machines. The cycle doesn't involve any impact, so it can be used for individuals who need to reduce the amount of impact to the joints, such as those with obesity or arthritis. As with the treadmill, the cycle can be used for either aerobic or anaerobic conditioning, depending on the intensity of the exercise. Steppers and rowers are also nonimpact machines that can be used for individuals wishing to avoid any impact on the joints, but it is important to remember that rowing can place a greater amount of stress on the lower back than other methods of cardiovascular exercise.

It is also recommended that information regarding health and safety is given to the individual during the induction session. Fire exits and emergency procedures can be pointed out, as well as water and toilet facilities. The

Table 13.3	Guidelines for cardiovascular equipment
Treadmill	**Foot action:** A heel–toe action should be encouraged when walking or jogging as this will help to absorb the shock of impact. At speeds around 8 mph, the client should be encouraged to use a midfoot strike as this will help to eliminate the braking effect. A two-degree grade increase makes the exercise comparable to walking/running outside **Arm action:** The most efficient way to swing the arms is with a 90-degree angle at the elbows and with the arms swinging close to the side of the body. Try to keep the shoulders relaxed at all times. **Posture:** Encourage the client to maintain a neutral spine with only a slight forward lean, which should increase slightly as the treadmill is inclined.
Cycle	**Seat height:** As the seat height can affect the range of motion and speed of the legs, it is important to make sure that the seat is level with the hip joint of the client when standing next to the cycle. With the client on the cycle and the feet flat in the pedals, the knee should have a slight bend at the furthest point of the rotation. **Pedal speed (cadence):** Actual pedal speed depends on the preference of the client. Most people prefer to pedal between 50 and 80 rpm, although this can increase during bouts of high intensity. **Posture:** Encourage an upright posture with neutral spine at all times. If using a recumbent cycle, encourage clients not to press their back flat into the seat and to try to maintain a neutral spine.
Stepper	**Range of motion:** With the whole of the foot placed on the step, encourage a full range of motion that is just before the end range of the machine. **Action:** As the leg raises during the stepping, the heel of the same leg should raise slightly off the pedal and return to the pedal as the leg goes down. **Speed:** Select a speed that is comfortable for the client. As the level on the step machine is increased, the resistance of the pedals will decrease, which means that the client will need to increase the speed. **Posture:** Encourage the client to hold the handles just to the side of the body rather than out in front. This will enable the client to maintain an upright posture with neutral spine.

Table 13.3	**Guidelines for cardiovascular equipment cont.**
Rower	**Start position (catch):** With the feet secured in the straps and the knees bent, hold the handle with a pronated grip (overhand) with the arms out straight and a slight bend at the elbows. Keep the wrists straight. The back should be in an upright neutral position.
	Drive: Initiate the drive phase with the legs pushing out. When the legs are almost at full stretch, pull the handle into the abdomen area.
	Recovery: The arms must extend fully before the legs bend to allow the body to come back to the start position. The recovery phase should be twice as long as the drive phase.

individual should also be made aware that they should terminate exercise at any time should they feel unwell or unable to continue.

NEED TO KNOW

The loss of balance that sometimes occurs when a treadmill comes to a stop is due to confusion in the brain, as the brain is used to objects in the distance becoming nearer when moving forward.

Resistance induction

Most beginners to resistance training are unfamiliar with the operation of resistance machines and free weights. It is therefore important to give clear explanations of how to operate resistance machines and the techniques involved in resistance training before the individual begins an exercise program.

As with the cardio induction, the instructor usually takes the individual through the resistance training session in order to establish intensity levels for the warm-up, main activity and cool-down. There are many methods of

inducting individuals in relation to resistance training, depending on the individual instructor's preference. However, in order to be consistent in the delivery, it is advisable to use a logical approach such as the NAMSIT method:

N	Name the machine or exercise
A	Area of the body working
M	Muscle group name
S	Silent demonstration
I	Instruct client to try
T	Teach the client

This approach can be used regardless of the resistance machine being used. It is important that instructors use good technique when demonstrating to prevent the individual copying 'bad' technique.

As with the cardiovascular demonstration, the visual demonstration for resistance exercises will provide a lot of information, so supplemetary verbal information should be kept to a minimum. When the individual is using the machine, the instructor should maintain a dialogue in order to give relevant information on performance and technique. The instructor should then aim to identify the suitable training intensity required for each resistance exercise.

Flexibility induction

As with any other part of the induction, it is important that the instructor provides a technically correct demonstration of all the stretches included in the exercise program. The gym environment should have a matted area for stretching. It is logical to start with standing stretches and then progress to seated stretches in order to decrease the heart rate progressively. Once the instructor has demonstrated the stretch, the individual should perform it. The instructor should then give feedback about the individual's technique and give instructions about the intensity and duration of the stretch.

TASK

Explain the two common methods of cardiovascular and resistance training induction, referring to their acronyms.

EXAMPLE QUESTIONS

13.1 According to the ACSM, what period of time is recommended for a warm-up?
   a) up to 5 minutes
   b) 5–10 minutes
   c) 10–20 minutes
   d) 20–60 minutes

13.2 According to the ACSM, what intensity of exercise, related to heart rate maximum, is recommended for the cardiovascular endurance component?
   a) 35–90 percent
   b) 45–90 percent
   c) 55–90 percent
   d) 65–90 percent

13.3 In relation to cardio training zones, what range of heart rate maximum is the weight-management zone?
   a) 50–60 percent
   b) 60–70 percent
   c) 70–80 percent
   d) 80–90 percent

13.4 In relation to cardio training zones, what range of heart rate maximum is the aerobic zone?
   a) 50–60 percent
   b) 60–70 percent
   c) 70–80 percent
   d) 80–90 percent

13.5 In relation to cardio training zones, what range of heart rate maximum is the anaerobic zone?
   a) 50–60 percent
   b) 60–70 percent
   c) 70–80 percent
   d) 80–90 percent

EXAMPLE QUESTIONS cont.

13.6 What type of training is otherwise known as 'speed play'?

   a) interval

   b) continuous

   c) intermittent

   d) fartlek

13.7 Which cycle of periodization is usually associated with a seven-day period?

   a) minicycle

   b) microcycle

   c) mesocycle

   d) macrocycle

13.8 Which cycle of periodization is usually associated with a period of a few weeks?

   a) minicycle

   b) microcycle

   c) mesocycle

   d) macrocycle

13.9 Which cycle of periodization is usually associated with a 12-month period?

   a) minicycle

   b) microcycle

   c) mesocycle

   d) macrocycle

13.10 What is the acronym NAMSIT used for?

   a) induction for cardiovascular machines

   b) induction for resistance machines

   c) the screening process

   d) risk stratification

EXAMPLE QUESTIONS cont.

13.11 What is the acronym IDEA used for?
   a) induction for cardiovascular machines
   b) induction for resistance machines
   c) the screening process
   d) risk stratification

13.12 Which of the following cardiovascular machines is normally associated with higher impact?
   a) cycle
   b) stepper
   c) treadmill
   d) rower

Further reading

American College of Sports Medicine (2006) *ACSM Guidelines to Exercise Testing and Prescription* (7th ed), Lippincott, Williams & Wilkins

Baechle, R.T. (2000) *Essentials of Strength Training and Conditioning*, Human Kinetics

Bompa, T.O. (1999) *Periodisation Training for Sports*, Human Kinetics

Bouchard, C., Shepard, R. and Stephens, T. (1994) *Physical Activity, Fitness and Health*, Human Kinetics

Howley, E.T. and Franks, B.D. (1997) *Health Fitness Instructor's Handbook* (3rd ed.), Human Kinetics

Marieb, E. (1998) *Human Anatomy and Physiology* (4th ed.), The Benjamin Cummings Publishing Company Inc.

McArdle, W.D., Katch, F.I. and Katch, V.L. (1996) *Exercise Physiology*, Lippincott, Williams & Wilkins

Sewell, D., Watkins, P. and Griffin, M. (2005) *Sport and Exercise Science: An Introduction*, Hodder Arnold

Tortora, G.J. and Grabowski, S.R. (2003) *Principles of Anatomy and Physiology* (10th ed.), Wiley

Wilmore, J.H. and Costhill, D.L. (2004) *Physiology of Sport and Exercise* (3rd ed.), Human Kinetics

Wilson, K.J.W. and Waugh, A. (1998) *Ross and Wilson Anatomy and Physiology in Health and Illness*, Churchill Livingstone

NOTES

MONITORING EXERCISE INTENSITY 14

OBJECTIVES

After completing this chapter, you will be able to

1 List and describe the cardiovascular training zones associated with the health and fitness industry.

2 Explain the various methods of monitoring cardiovascular and resistance exercise intensity.

3 Calculate percentages of heart rate maximum.

Instructing Exercise and Fitness Knowledge

Basic Anatomy and Physiology
- Exercises that are safe and appropriate for participants.
- How to plan to use a range of cardiovascular and resistance machines and weights.

Instructing Physical Activity and Exercise Knowledge

Energy Systems and Components of Fitness
- Heart-rate training zones
- Metabolic equivalents
- Monitoring exercise intensity:
  - Rate of perceived exertion, talk test, lactic testing, heart rate monitoring
  - Benefits and limitations of each method

Introduction

This chapter deals with common methods of prescribing and monitoring exercise intensity employed within the health and fitness industry. Instructors should be able to list the common methods of monitoring cardiovascular and resistance exercise intensity and explain each within the context of the health and fitness industry.

Other chapters in the book provide information regarding the practical application of the theoretical content, which, along with the information covered in this chapter, will provide instructors with the understanding and ability to design appropriate exercise programs for apparently healthy individuals, in line with current guidelines for exercise.

Exercise intensity

Intensity refers to the difficulty level of a particular exercise or, in simple terms, how hard the exercise feels to the individual. When designing an exercise program, instructors can prescribe intensity levels that best suit the individual's goals. For example an individual might have weight loss and toning as goals. In this case the instructor could set cardiovascular intensity within the weight-management training zone and resistance training intensity at around 10–12 repetition max (RM) (see Chapter 10).

Monitoring the intensity level at which an individual is exercising can also help instructors to adjust the exercise program accordingly. Monitoring can give the instructor information regarding fitness progression or any drop in performance that might indicate signs of overtraining, allowing them to use this information to make necessary adjustments to the program.

When prescribing exercise at a specific intensity, it is useful to understand the physiology in relation to each component of fitness (see Chapter 10). Intensity levels of both cardiovascular exercise and resistance exercise can be monitored in several different ways. Monitoring intensity within a health and fitness environment is not as accurate as monitoring within a laboratory environment but is still useful if the lack of accuracy is taken into consideration.

Monitoring cardiovascular intensity

Several methods can be used to prescribe and monitor a particular cardiovascular exercise intensity for an individual, including heart rate, metabolic equivalents, self-perception (METs) (rate of perceived exertion [RPE]) and communication skills (the talk test).

Heart rate

One of the most common methods of prescribing or monitoring cardiovascular intensity is the heart rate method. As the intensity of the exercise increases, the heart rate of the individual increases in a linear fashion. It therefore follows that as training zones are related to a percentage of maximum heart rate (see pages 196–97), the percentage of maximum heart rate that has been agreed for the exercise can be related to the goals of the individual. For example, if the individual wants to develop aerobic fitness, he or she should exercise at a heart rate level of 70–80 percent of their maximum (the aerobic zone). This can be written as 70–80%HRM.

Two steps need to be taken in order to convert the chosen percentage of heart rate maximum into beats per minute. First, the maximum heart rate of the individual needs to be found; second, the required percentage of this maximum needs to be calculated.

Step 1: Calculating the maximum heart rate for an individual.

Maximum heart rate can be calculated by using one of two methods: one way is to carry out a maximum graded heart rate test, and the other is to use a formula for predicting maximum heart rate.

Maximum graded heart rate test

Several tests are available in which intensity is increased until the point at which there is no rise in heart rate, even though the intensity is continuing to increase. This type of test is reasonably accurate but is not suitable for any individual who is tested within the health and fitness environment as National Occupational Standards guidelines recommend that instructors advise exercise intensity only up to a maximum of 90 percent of heart rate maximum.

Predicted maximum heart rate

As an alternative to a maximum graded heart rate test, the following formula can be used to predict maximum heart rate:

$$\text{Maximum heart rate} = 220 - \text{age}$$

For example, a 23-year-old person would have a predicted maximum heart rate of 197 bpm (220 – 23 = 197) and a 45-year-old person would have a predicted maximum heart rate of 175 bpm (220 – 45). Even though there are errors associated with this method of estimating maximum heart rate (there can be an error of plus or minus 12 bpm using this method), it is commonly used and is suitable for the health and fitness industry.

Step 2: Calculating the percentage of the maximum heart rate in bpm

Once the maximum heart rate has been established, it is possible to calculate the percentage of heart rate maximum that is required for the individual in beats per minute (bpm): the maximum heart rate for the individual is multiplied by the chosen percentage. For instance, a 32-year-old individual needs to perform the exercise at 70–80 percent of maximum heart rate (the aerobic zone). The instructor should calculate the individual's training intensity heart rates at 70 and 80 percent of maximum as follows:

1. Predicted maximum heart rate for the individual is 220 – age (32) = 188 bpm
2. 70 percent of maximum (188 bpm) = 188/100 × 70 = 131 bpm
3. 80 percent of maximum (188 bpm) = (188/100 × 80) = 150 bpm

Note: Round the answer to the nearest whole number.

Therefore, in order to exercise at the desired intensity, the individual would need to keep their heart rate between 131 and 150 bpm. Over a period of time, if the individual could maintain this heart rate but at an increased speed, this would indicate that the individual was becoming fitter. This is one method of monitoring cardiovascular fitness.

Metabolic equivalents

The intensity of an exercise can be linked to the amount of energy expended by the individual: the greater the intensity level of the exercise, the greater the energy expenditure required to sustain that level. A *MET* is a way of expressing expenditure in either calories (kcal) or volume of oxygen (VO_2). The resting value of 1 MET is expressed as follows:

$$1 \text{ MET} = 3.5 \text{ mlO}_2.\text{kg}^{-1}\text{min}^{-1} \text{ or } 1\text{kcal.kg}^{-1}\text{hr}^{-1}$$

It follows that an exercise that requires four times as much energy than that used at rest would have a value of 4 METs and an exercise that requires 10 times as much would have a value of 10 METs, and so on. Even though MET values are commonly shown on cardiovascular machines, the use of METs seems to be restricted to medical use for exercise prescription. If the machines

Table 14.1	Metabolic equivalents (METs) for various activities
Activities between 3 and 6 METs	**Activities more than 6 METs**
Housework:	**Housework:**
Polishing	Any heavy housework
Cleaning windows	Any heavy gardening
Making beds	
Mopping floors	**Activities:**
Vacuuming	Jogging
Hanging washing	Running
Sweeping	Brisk cycling
Gardening – light work	Brisk swimming
	Wheeling in wheelchair
Activities:	High-impact aerobics
Slow walking	Martial arts
Brisk walking	Circuit training
Slow cycling	Skipping
Slow swimming	
Skating	**Sports:**
Gentle aerobics	Dancing
Yoga	Tennis
Dancing (ballroom etc.)	Horse riding
Golf	Squash
Table tennis	Basketball
	Football
	Gymnastics
Sports:	Fencing
Fencing	Skiing
Archery	Rugby
Cricket	Netball
	Boxing

Note: This table has been adapted from a variety of sources and should be used as an approximation of metabolic equivalent values related to various activities.

used do not display MET values, there are many published tables that estimate them for a range of activities (see Table 14.1). These activities can extend to household chores and outdoor activities as well as fitness facility activities.

As METs have a value expressed in calories, if the weight of the individual is known then the amount of calories expended during a particular exercise can also be calculated. Take, for example, a 75 kg person exercising at 10 METs for one hour:

10 METs = 10 kcals per kilo of bodyweight every hour, and 10 (kcals) × 75 (kg) = 750. Therefore, this person would expend 750 kcals.

NEED TO KNOW

Any activities between 3 and 6 METs are considered moderate-intensity physical activity. Any activities greater than 6 METs are considered vigorous-intensity physical activity.

Rate of perceived exertion

Another method of setting and monitoring the appropriate exercise intensity for an individual is to use the *RPE* scale (see Table 14.2), which was first introduced by Dr. Gunnar Borg and is sometimes known as the Borg scale.

The RPE scale is a method of measuring the subjective feelings of an individual during exercise. The individual's perception of the level of difficulty during cardiovascular exercise has been found to correlate very strongly with heart rate. For this reason, the RPE scale is widely used as an alternative to heart rate.

Two different scales are commonly used: the 6–20 scale and the revised 0–10+ scale, also known as the *category ratio* or *CR-10 scale*. The individual is shown the scale during exercise and asked how he or she feels compared with the words on the scale. This perception is then used to estimate either the percentage of heart rate maximum or the heart rate. For example, if the individual states that the exercise feels 'somewhat hard,' this equates to level 13 on the 6–20 scale, which corresponds to approximately 130 bpm or 70 percent of maximum heart rate. Depending on the goals of the individual, the instructor can recommend an RPE level at which to exercise without the need to monitor heart rate.

Even though the subjective perception of exercise intensity correlates well with heart rate, it is important to note that various individuals carrying out exactly the same exercise session might report different levels of RPE. There are many factors that could affect this perception rating, such as fitness levels, exercise familiarity and illness.

NEED TO KNOW

Research has shown that perception rating on the 6–20 scale correlates closely with heart rate: for example a 'very light' rating equates to 9 on the scale, which would be a heart rate of approximately 90 bpm.

Talk test

Although the talk test is not a particularly scientific method of determining cardiovascular exercise intensity, it can be used as an alternative to heart rate, METs or RPE due to the ease of administration. The talk test is simply a matter of talking to the individual during exercise and gauging the level of intensity from the response of the individual. If the individual is able to carry out a normal conversation, this usually indicates that they are in either the weight-management zone or the lower end of the aerobic zone (see pages 196–97). If the

Table 14.2	Rate of perceived exertion (Borg) scale	
6–20 scale	**0–10 scale**	**Estimate of %MHR**
6	0 Nothing at all	
7 Very, very light	0.3	
8	0.5 Extremely weak	50%
9 Very light	0.7	55%
10	1 Very weak	60%
11 Fairly light	1.5	65%
12	2 Weak	70%
13 Somewhat hard	2.5	75%
14	3 Moderate	80%
15 Hard	4	85%
16	5 Strong	88%
17 Very hard	6	92%
18	7 Very strong	96%
19 Very, very hard	8	98%
20	9	100%
	10 Extremely strong	
	11	
	Absolute maximum	

Adapted from *ACSM Guidelines for Exercise Testing and Prescription* (2006).
Key: MHR = maximum heart rate

individual becomes breathless and has difficulty maintaining a normal conversation, this usually means they are in the anaerobic zone. The instructor can then adjust the level of intensity accordingly, depending on the goal of the exercise session.

Once the required level of intensity of a cardiovascular exercise session has been attained using the talk test method, the instructor can empower the individual to take responsibility for maintaining that level in subsequent exercise sessions. The individual should be informed that they can progress by increasing the intensity of the exercise as long as they are still able to carry out a normal conversation.

TASK

List the methods of monitoring cardiovascular intensity and briefly describe how each method is used.

Monitoring resistance intensity

When prescribing the intensity of a resistance exercise (how heavy the weight should be), the instructor can use a percentage of the maximum capability of that individual, known as 1RM (see page 153). However, one disadvantage of this method is that the maximum capability of the individual must be found before a percentage of this can be calculated. As the individual would have to perform to maximum capability, the risk of injury would be high and not in line with recommended guidelines (see page 155).

An easier method would be to use a multiple of the RM, such as 10RM or 15RM, which means the maximum weight the individual can lift 10 or 15 times, respectively. The ACSM guidelines for strength and endurance are given in multiples of RM. For example, in order to gain strength it is recommended that an individual performs resistance exercise using weights within the range of 8–12RM and to improve endurance using weights within the range of 10–15RM. Research has shown that the multiple of RM correlates to a percentage of the maximum capability (see Table 14.3).

Calculating repetition maximum

When trying to establish the amount of weight an individual can lift for a specific number of repetitions (RM), a certain procedure should be used to ensure that the individual is sufficiently warmed in order to minimize the risk of injury. If the instructor and the individual have agreed that an intensity of 12RM is going to be used for a particular exercise, the individual should first perform 12 repetitions of a known light weight.

Table 14.3	Repetition maximum compared with percentage of maximum capability	
Repetition maximum	% of maximum capability
1	100.0
2	93.5
3	91.0
4	88.5
5	86.0
6	83.5
7	81.0
8	78.5
9	76.0

Adapted from Baechle (2000).

Then add more weight depending on the ease of the first set and have the individual perform another 12 repetitions. Repeat this process until the individual can perform 12 repetitions only, and not 13. Ensure that sufficient rest is given between sets to recover: two to three minutes should be sufficient. The final weight (or load) that the individual could lift 12 times, and not 13, is the 12RM for that particular exercise. This process should then be repeated for all the exercises in the resistance training program.

For progression purposes (and assuming that the multiple RM chosen is to remain constant), when the individual is capable of comfortably performing the chosen RM, the weight can be increased by a small amount. If the individual cannot perform the number of chosen repetitions at the increased weight, they must revert to the original weight. This type of in-built progression is easy to implement, and as such, the instructor should empower the individual to take control of monitoring their own progression.

TASK

Briefly describe the term 'repetition maximum' and explain how it is used to determine the intensity of the resistance exercise to be performed.

EXAMPLE QUESTIONS

14.1 What is the formula for predicted maximum heart rate?
   a) 200 – age
   b) 210 – age
   c) 220 – age
   d) 230 – age

14.2 True or false? Predicted maximum heart rate has an error of up to plus or minus 12 beats per minute.
   True
   False

14.3 True or false? A graded maximum heart rate test should be used on all individuals to find their maximum heart rate.
   True
   False

14.4 What is the predicted maximum heart rate for a 39-year-old person?
   a) 171 bpm
   b) 181 bpm
   c) 179 bpm
   d) 189 bpm

14.5 What is 70 percent of the predicted maximum heart rate for a 20-year-old person?
   a) 120 bpm
   b) 130 bpm
   c) 140 bpm
   d) 150 bpm

14.6 What is 80 percent of the predicted maximum heart rate for a 40-year-old person?
   a) 144 bpm
   b) 154 bpm
   c) 138 bpm
   d) 148 bpm

EXAMPLE QUESTIONS cont.

14.7 What is 55 percent of the predicted maximum heart rate for a 40-year-old person?
a) 89 bpm
b) 92 bpm
c) 95 bpm
d) 99 bpm

14.8 What is the equivalent value of 1 MET?
a) 1.5 $mlO_2.kg^{-1}min^{-1}$
b) 2.5 $mlO_2.kg^{-1}min^{-1}$
c) 3.5 $mlO_2.kg^{-1}min^{-1}$
d) 4.5 $mlO_2.kg^{-1}min^{-1}$

14.9 What is the equivalent value of 1 MET?
a) 1.0 $kcal.kg^{-1}hr^{-1}$
b) 1.5 $kcal.kg^{-1}hr^{-1}$
c) 2.0 $kcal.kg^{-1}hr^{-1}$
d) 2.5 $kcal.kg^{-1}hr^{-1}$

14.10 How many kilocalories would an 80 kg person expend in 30 minutes doing an exercise valued at 10 METs?
a) 350
b) 400
c) 450
d) 500

14.11 How many kilocalories would a 60 kg person expend in two hours and 30 minutes doing an exercise valued at 8 METs?
a) 1,000
b) 1,100
c) 1,200
d) 1,400

EXAMPLE QUESTIONS cont.

14.12 Which of the following statements is most accurate in regard to the definition of 12RM?
a) A weight that can be easily lifted 12 times
b) A weight at which the performer fails on the 12th repetition
c) A weight that can be lifted at least 12 times
d) A weight that can be lifted 12 times and not 13 times

Further reading

American College of Sports Medicine (2006) *ACSM Guidelines for Exercise Testing and Prescription* (7th ed.), Lippincott, Williams & Wilkins

Baechle, R.T. (2000) *Essentials of Strength Training and Conditioning*, Human Kinetics

Bouchard, C., Shepard, R. and Stephens, T. (1994) *Physical Activity, Fitness and Health*, Human Kinetics

Howley, E.T. and Franks, B.D. (1997) *Health Fitness Instructors Handbook* (3rd ed.), Human Kinetics

Marieb, E. (1998) *Human Anatomy and Physiology* (4th ed.), The Benjamin Cummings Publishing Company Inc.

McArdle, W.D., Katch, F.I. and Katch, V.L. (1996) *Exercise Physiology*, Lippincott, Williams & Wilkins

Sewell, D., Watkins, P. and Griffin, M. (2005) *Sport and Exercise Science: An Introduction*, Hodder Arnold

Tortora, G.J. and Grabowski, S.R. (2003) *Principles of Anatomy and Physiology* (10th ed.), Wiley

Wilmore, J.H. and Costhill, D.L. (2004) *Physiology of Sport and Exercise* (3rd ed.), Human Kinetics

Wilson, K.J.W. and Waugh, A. (1998) *Ross and Wilson Anatomy and Physiology in Health and Illness*, Churchill Livingstone

NOTES

FREE-WEIGHT AND RESISTANCE MACHINE EXERCISES

OBJECTIVES

After completing this chapter, the reader should be able to

1   List and describe common free-weight and resistance machine exercises associated with the health and fitness industry.

2   Describe how each exercise is carried out in terms of technique.

3   List the major muscles and synergists responsible for the exercises.

4   Give alternatives for each exercise.

Instructing Exercise and Fitness Knowledge

Basic Anatomy and Physiology

- Exercises that are safe and appropriate for participants.

- How to plan to use a range of cardiovascular and resistance machines, weights.

- The effect of speed on posture, alignment and intensity.

- The effect of levers, gravity and resistance on the exercise.

- A range of resistance machines, weights, barbells, dumbbells, collars, benches, protective floor mats.

- The safe storage of free-weight equipment.

- Safe manual handling techniques.

Introduction

This chapter deals with common free-weight and resistance machine exercises employed within the health and fitness industry. Instructors should be able to list the common resistance exercises and the major muscles used in each. Instructors should also be able to describe how to perform and give alternatives to each exercise.

This chapter builds upon the information in other chapters of this book, regarding the practical application of the theoretical content, to provide the instructor with an understanding of the correct performance technique associated with a range of free-weight and resistance machine exercises.

Free-weight and resistance exercises

The choice of performing resistance exercises using free weights or machines is an individual preference. However, there are several issues that are common within the health and fitness environment (see Table 15.1).

The examples of free-weight and resistance machine exercises given in this chapter are typical of those used by beginners to this type of training. There are many other exercises common to the health and fitness environment, which can be considered to be more advanced or for those with at least several months experience of weight training. It is crucial that all beginners to resistance exercises are shown the correct technique in a demonstration prior to performing the exercise themselves. Beginners must also be shown safety-related points, such as how to attach collars to weight-lifting bars, how to pick up and return free weights from their storage racks and how to keep the exercise area clear of obstructions. As research is sparse in relation to musculoskeletal injury as a consequence of resistance training, the following examples describe how to perform each exercise with what is considered to be safe technique within the health and fitness industry. The major and synergistic muscles (see Chapter 3) for each exercise are also listed, along with alternatives for each exercise that involve the same muscle groups.

Table 15.1	Health and fitness issues
Issue	Comment
Type of equipment	**Barbell** A long bar with weights attached at either end for use with both hands. **Dumbbell** A small bar with weights attached at either end for use with one hand only. **Collars** These are used on barbells and dumbbells to prevent the weights coming off. They must be used at all times with free weights. **Benches** Make sure benches are robust enough to use with free weights. **Floor mats** These are recommended in the area where free weights are used to prevent damage to the floor and the weights.

Table 15.1	Health and fitness issues cont.
Speed of execution	All exercises must be performed under control so that muscles are worked through their full range and posture is not compromised.
Range of movement	Always use the full range of movement possible for each exercise. Try to keep the repetitions continuous rather than rest at either the start or midpoint.
Breathing	A breath out is normally done during the exertion of the exercise. If this is confusing, just breathe normally.
Alignment	Neutral posture must be maintained during all exercises.
Storage	Return free weights to their storage racks after use.
Handling technique	When lifting free weights from the floor, adopt a squat position and keep the weights close to the body.
Levers	To increase the intensity of the exercise, take weights further from the body (increase lever length).
Gravity	For free weights to be effective the weight must travel in a vertical direction.

Chest Press

Major muscles used: pectoralis major

Synergist muscles used: anterior deltoid, tricep, serratus anterior

- Make sure the feet are placed firmly on the ground and that the upper arms are parallel to the floor (Figure 15.1).
- The palms should be facing forward and the hands should be directly above the elbows.
- Raise the weights in an arcing motion, keeping them in line with the chest until the arms are fully extended.

Awareness points:
Keep the hands directly above the elbows at all times and make sure that the wrists remain firm. Lower the weights under control until the upper arms are parallel with the floor. Maintain a normal lumbar curve at all times.

Alternatives: machine chest press, chest fly, pec dec, push-up.

Figure 15.1 **(a) and (b): Chest press**

(a) Start position

(b) Midposition

Chest Fly

Major muscles used: pectoralis major

Synergist muscles used: anterior deltoid, serratus anterior

- Make sure the feet are placed firmly on the ground and that the upper arms are parallel to the floor.
- Do not extend the arms fully. Maintain a slight flexion at the elbow joint with the palms facing upward.
- Bring the weights together in an arcing motion, keeping them in line with the chest.

Awareness points: Avoid fully extending the arms at all times. Lower the weights under control until the upper arms are parallel with the floor. Maintain a normal lumbar curve at all times.

Alternatives: chest press, pec dec, push-up.

Figure 15.2 **(a) and (b): Chest fly**

(a) Start position

(b) Midposition

Single-Arm Row

Major muscles used: latissimus dorsi

Synergist muscles used: bicep brachialis, posterior deltoid

- Adopt a kneeling position with one leg so that the hip joint of that leg is approximately 90 degrees and the supporting hand is directly below the shoulder.
- Place the supporting leg on the ground slightly away from the bench but at the level of the hip joint.
- Fully extend the arm while holding the weight with the palm turned inward.
- Draw the weight toward the hip joint until the upper arm is parallel with the floor.

Awareness points: Keep the head facing down to maintain neutral cervical spine. Maintain a normal lumbar curve at all times.

Alternatives: lat pull down, seated row

Figure 15.3 (a) and (b): Single-arm row

(a) Start position

(b) Midposition

Shoulder Press

Major muscles used: deltoids (anterior, medial and posterior)

Synergist muscles used: tricep

- Stand with feet shoulder-width apart and the spine in neutral position. Ensure upper arms are slightly below parallel position with hands directly above the elbow joint.
- The palms should be facing forward and in line with the front of the face.
- Raise the weights in an arcing motion, keeping them in line with the front of the face until the arms are fully extended.

Awareness points: Both hands should remain within peripheral vision at all times. Maintain a normal lumbar curve at all times.

Alternatives: machine shoulder press, lateral raise, upright row

Figure 15.4 (a) and (b): Shoulder press

(a) Start position

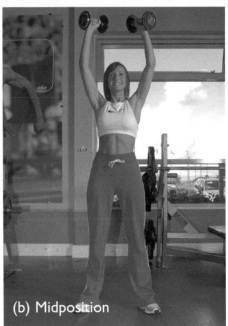

(b) Midposition

Lateral Raise

Major muscles used: deltoids (anterior, medial and posterior)

Synergist muscles used: trapezius (upper fibers during shoulder elevation)

- Stand with feet shoulder-width apart and the spine in neutral position. Hang arms by the sides with a slight bend at the elbow joint so that the weight is slightly forward of the hip joint, palms facing inward.
- Raise the weights in an abduction motion, keeping them in line and slightly forward of the hip joint until the arms are parallel to the floor.

Awareness points: Both hands should remain within peripheral vision at all times. Maintain a normal lumbar curve at all times. Stop when the arms are parallel to the floor to avoid impingement at the acromioclavicular joint.

Alternatives: shoulder press, upright row

Figure 15.5 **(a) and (b): Lateral raise**

(a) Start position

(b) Midposition

Upright Row

Major muscles used: deltoids (anterior, medial and posterior)

Synergist muscles used: trapezius (upper fibers during shoulder elevation), bicep brachialis

- Stand with feet shoulder-width apart and the spine in neutral position. Hang arms to the front of the body with a slight bend at the elbow joint, palms facing inward.
- Raise the weights in a vertical motion, keeping them in front of the body until the upper arms are parallel to the floor.

Awareness points: Maintain a normal lumbar curve at all times. Stop when the upper arms are parallel to the floor to avoid impingement at the acromioclavicular joint.

Alternatives: lateral raise, shoulder press

Figure 15.6 **(a) and (b): Upright row**

(a) Start position

(b) Midposition

Overhead Tricep Extension

Major muscles used: tricep

Synergist muscles used: anconeus

- Stand with feet shoulder-width apart and spine in neutral position. Extend upper arm directly above the head with a 90-degree bend at the elbow, palm facing inward.
- Palm facing inward.
- Extend the arm so that the hand is directly above the shoulder joint.

Awareness points: Maintain a normal lumbar curve at all times. Make sure that the weight remains to the side of the head at all times.

Alternatives: tricep push-down, tricep kick-back, narrow-arm push-up.

Figure 15.7 **(a) and (b): Tricep extension**

(a) Start position

(b) Midposition

Tricep Kick-back

Major muscles used: tricep

Synergist muscles used: anconeus

- Adopt a kneeling position with one leg so that the hip joint of that leg is at approximately 90 degrees and the supporting hand is directly below the shoulder.
- Place the supporting leg on the ground slightly away from the bench but at the level of the hip joint.
- With the palm turned inward raise the upper arm until it is parallel with the floor and keep a 90-degree angle at the elbow joint.
- Extend the lower arm backward until it is parallel with the floor.

Awareness points: Keep the head facing down to maintain neutral cervical spine. Maintain a normal lumbar curve at all times.

Alternatives: tricep push-down, tricep extension, narrow-arm push-up.

Figure 15.8 (a) and (b): Tricep kick-back

(a) Start position

(b) Midposition

Bicep Curl

Major muscles used: biceps brachii

Synergist muscles used: bicep brachialis, brachioradialis

- Stand with feet shoulder-width apart and spine in neutral position. Hang arms by the sides with palms facing forward.
- Raise the weights in a line toward the face as if feeding.

Awareness points: Maintain a normal lumbar curve at all times. Make sure that the weights do not strike the face and lower them to full extension of the elbow joint.

Alternative: bicep curl machine

Figure 15.9 (a) and (b): Bicep curl

(a) Start position

(b) Midposition

Squat

Major muscles used: quadriceps, hamstrings, gluteus maximus, erector spinae

Synergist muscles used: Some of the muscles above work as synergists depending on the angle of the torso

- Stand with feet shoulder-width apart and spine in neutral position. Hang arms by the sides with palms facing inward.
- Bend the hip joint and knee joint as in a sitting motion until the thighs are approximately parallel with the floor.

Awareness points: Maintain a normal lumbar curve at all times. The head should drop and raise in a vertical line so that the body does not tilt forward.

Alternatives: squat machine, leg press

Figure 15.10 **(a) and (b): Squat**

(a) Start position

(b) Midposition

Chest Press

Major muscles used: pectoralis major

Synergist muscles used: anterior deltoid, tricep, serratus anterior

- Make sure feet are placed firmly on the ground and that the seat is at the height where the arms are parallel to the floor.
- The upper arms should be in line with the body.
- Fully extend the arms, keeping the wrists firm.

Awareness points: Maintain a normal lumbar curve at all times. Do not allow the hands to go out of peripheral vision at any time.

Alternatives: free-weight chest press, chest fly, pec dec, push-ups

Figure 15.11 **(a) and (b): Chest press**

(a) Start position

(b) Midposition

Pec Dec

Major muscles used: pectoralis major

Synergist muscles used: anterior deltoid, serratus anterior

- Make sure the feet are placed firmly on the ground and that the seat is at the height where the upper arms are parallel to the floor.
- The arms should be in line with the body.
- Bring the arms together under control.

Awareness points: Maintain a normal lumbar curve at all times. Do not allow the hands to go out of peripheral vision at any time.

Alternatives: chest press, chest fly, push-ups

Figure 15.12   (a) and (b): Pec dec

(a) Start position

(b) Midposition

Shoulder Press

Major muscles used: deltoids (anterior, medial and posterior)

Synergist muscles used: tricep

- Make sure feet are firmly on the ground and the spine is in neutral position. Adjust the seat height until the upper arms are slightly below parallel position.
- Raise the arms until they are fully extended.

Awareness points: Both hands should remain within peripheral vision at all times. Maintain a normal lumbar curve at all times.

Alternatives: free-weight shoulder press, lateral raise, upright row

Figure 15.13 **(a) and (b): Shoulder press**

(a) Start position

(b) Midposition

Seated Row

Major muscles used: latissimus dorsi

Synergist muscles used: bicep brachialis, posterior deltoid, rhomboids

- Make sure feet are firmly on the floor and the spine is in a neutral position.
- The chest support should be adjusted so that the hands can take a firm grip of the handles with the chest on the support.
- Adjust the seat height so that the arms are roughly parallel to the floor.
- Draw the weight toward the body until the upper arm is parallel with the plane of the body.

Awareness points: Keep the head facing forward to maintain neutral cervical spine. Maintain a normal lumbar curve at all times. Only draw the upper arms back to the plane of the body to avoid undue strain on the trapezius muscle.

Alternatives: lat pull-down, single-arm row

Figure 15.14 (a) and (b): Seated row

(a) Start position

(b) Midposition

Lat Pull-down

Major muscles used: latissimus dorsi

Synergist muscles used: bicep brachialis, posterior deltoid

- Make sure the feet are firmly on the floor and the spine is in a neutral position.
- Adjust the seat height so that the arms are almost at full extension when gripping the handles on the bar.
- Draw it vertically down in front of the body until the bar is roughly in line with the chin level.

Awareness points: Keep the head facing forward to maintain neutral cervical spine. Maintain a normal lumbar curve at all times. Only draw the bar to chin level to avoid undue strain on the rotator cuff muscles. Draw the bar to the front of the body to avoid stress on the shoulder joints.

Alternatives: seated row, single-arm row

Figure 15.15 | **(a) and (b): Lat pull-down**

(a) Start position

(b) Midposition

Back Extension

Major muscles used: most of the erector spinae group of muscles

Synergist muscles used: Multifidus and some of the many individual muscles that make up the erector spinae group

- Make sure feet are firmly on the floor or foot plate and the spine is in a neutral position.
- Place the pad across the shoulder level with the torso in a flexed position.
- Extend the back to a position where the spine is in neutral.

Awareness points: Keep the head facing forward to maintain neutral cervical spine. Maintain a normal lumbar curve at all times. Avoid going into extension of the spine.

Alternatives: free-weight squat, dorsal raise

Figure 15.16 (a) and (b): Back extension

(a) Start position

(b) Midposition

Abdominal Crunch

Major muscles used: rectus abdominis

Synergist muscles used: hip flexors, external and internal obliques

- Make sure feet are firmly on the floor and the spine is in a neutral position.
- Place the pad across the upper chest.
- Draw the torso toward the knees.

Awareness points: Keep the head facing forward to maintain neutral cervical spine. Maintain a normal lumbar curve at all times.

Alternatives: sit-ups, crunches

Figure 15.17	(a) and (b): Abdominal crunch

(a) Start position

(b) Midposition

Tricep Push-down

Major muscles used: tricep

Synergist muscles used: anconeus

- Make sure feet are shoulder-width apart and the spine is in a neutral position. Grip the bar shoulder-width apart so that the upper arms are just forward of the body line, palm facing downward.
- Extend the upper and lower arm so that the arms are both fully straight.

Awareness points: Maintain a normal lumbar curve at all times.

Alternatives: tricep extension, tricep kick-back, narrow-arm push-up.

Figure 15.18 (a) and (b): Tricep push-down

(a) Start position

(b) Midposition

Bicep Curl

Major muscles used: bicep brachii

Synergist muscles used: bicep brachialis, brachioradialis

- Make sure the feet are shoulder-width apart and the spine is in a neutral position. Grip the handles so that the upper arms are on the pads and the palms face upward.
- Bring the handles toward the face until the elbow joint is fully flexed.

Awareness points: Maintain a normal lumbar curve at all times. Keep the upper arms on the pad at all times. Fully extend the arms on the downward phase.

Alternative: free-weight bicep curl

Figure 15.19 (a) and (b): Bicep curl

(a) Start position

(b) Midposition

Seated Adductor

Major muscles used: adductor longus brevis and magnus, gracilis, pectinius

- Ensure the feet are firmly on the foot plates and the pads are on the inside of the knees.
- Use the machine setting to open the legs to a comfortable starting position.
- Bring the legs together against the resistance.

Awareness points: Maintain a normal lumbar curve at all times. Keep the knees and the toes pointing directly upward at all times.

Alternatives: squats, leg press, lunges, multi-hip machine

Figure 15.20 **(a) and (b): Seated adductor**

(a) Start position

(b) Midposition

Seated Abductor

Major muscles used: gluteus minimus and maximus

Synergist muscles used: tensor fascia latae

- Make sure the feet are firmly on the foot plates and the pads are on the outside of the knees.
- Use the machine setting to start with the legs together.
- Open the legs outward against the resistance.

Awareness points: Maintain a normal lumbar curve at all times. Open the legs to a full range of motion.

Alternatives: squats, leg press, lunges, multi-hip machine

Figure 15.21 **(a) and (b): Seated abductor**

(a) Start position

(b) Midposition

Leg Extension

Major muscles used: quadriceps

- Place the roller pads just above the ankle joint.
- Use the machine seat-setting to move the seat so that the knee joint aligns with the axis of the machine.
- Start with the knees flexed as far as comfortably possible.
- Extend the knees to full range of motion.

Awareness points: Maintain a normal lumbar curve at all times. Keep the knees and the toes pointing directly upward at all times. Ensure that full extension is achieved.

Alternatives: squats, leg press, lunges

Figure 15.22	(a) and (b): Leg extension

(a) Start position

(b) Midposition

Seated Leg Curl

Major muscles used: hamstrings

Synergist muscles used: calf

- Place the roller pads just above the calcaneus or heel bone.
- Use the machine seat-setting to move the seat so that the knee joint aligns with the axis of the machine.
- Start with the knees extended as far as comfortably possible.
- Flex the knees to full range of motion.

Awareness points: Maintain a normal lumbar curve at all times. Keep the knees and the toes pointing directly upward at all times.

Alternatives: squats, leg press, lunges

Figure 15.23	(a) and (b): Seated leg curl

(a) Start position

(b) Midposition

Leg Press

Major muscles used: quadriceps, hamstrings, gluteus maximus.

Synergist muscles used: Some of the muscles above work as synergists depending on the foot placement

- Place the feet about hip-width apart on the foot plate.
- Use the machine seat-setting to move the seat so that the knee joint is flexed to the maximum comfortable position.
- Extend the knees to full range of motion.

Awareness points: Maintain a normal lumbar curve at all times. Keep the knees and the toes in line at all times. Ensure that full extension at the knee joint is achieved.

Alternatives: squats, lunges

Figure 15.24 **(a) and (b): Leg press**

(a) Start position

(b) Midposition

EXAMPLE QUESTIONS: ANSWERS FOR REVIEW

I The skeletal system

1.1 The ulna is an example of which type of bone?

  a) Long bone

1.2 The patella is an example of which type of bone?

  d) Sesamoid bone

1.3 The pelvis is an example of which type of bone?

  c) Flat bone

1.4 What is the name for the shaft of a long bone?

  b) Diaphysis

1.5 Which two regions of the spine are primary curves?

  c) Thoracic and sacrum

1.6 Which two regions of the spine are secondary curves?

  d) Lumbar and cervical

1.7 Tendons attach to a layer of tissue covering a bone. What is this covering called?

  d) Periosteum

1.8 What are the cells in the bone that are responsible for bone-building called?

  b) Osteoblast cells

1.9 What are the cells in the bone that are responsible for breaking down bone called?

  c) Osteoclast cells

EXAMPLE QUESTIONS: ANSWERS FOR REVIEW cont.

1.10 Which two regions of the spine are capable of the most movement?

   d) Lumbar and cervical

1.11 What is the outer part of an intervertebral disk called?

   a) Annulus fibrosus

1.12 What is the inner part of an intervertebral disk called?

   b) Nucleus pulposus

 NOTES

EXAMPLE QUESTIONS: ANSWERS FOR REVIEW

2 Joints

2.1 The tibia and the fibula make what type of joint?

a) fixed

2.2 The pelvis and the sacrum make what type of joint?

a) fixed

2.3 The pelvis and the femur make what type of joint?

c) synovial

2.4 The atlas and the axis make what type of joint?

b) cartilaginous

2.5 Which of the following is classed as a hinge joint?

c) ankle

2.6 Which two movements are available at a hinge joint?

b) flexion and extension

2.7 Which of the following make a joint?

c) sacrum and coccyx

2.8 Which of the following make a joint?

b) ulna and radius

2.9 Which of the following make a joint?

a) humerus and ulna

EXAMPLE QUESTIONS: ANSWERS FOR REVIEW cont.

2.10 Which of the following make a joint?

a) tibia and fibula

2.11 Which of the following makes a gliding joint?

d) bones of the carpals

2.12 Which of the following makes a pivot joint?

b) ulna and radius

 NOTES

EXAMPLE QUESTIONS: ANSWERS FOR REVIEW

3 The muscular system

3.1 What is the main fuel of slow-twitch fibers?

a) fat and oxygen

3.2 What is the main fuel of fast-twitch fibers?

c) glucose

3.3 Which type of muscle can be found in arteries?

d) smooth

3.4 Which type of muscle can be found in the heart?

b) cardiac

3.5 In muscle contraction, which neurotransmitter stimulates the release of calcium?

b) acetylcholine

3.6 What is the name for the type of contraction when the muscle lengthens?

c) eccentric

3.7 What is the name for the type of contraction when the muscle shortens?

b) concentric

3.8 What is the name for a muscle that opposes the prime mover?

d) antagonist

3.9 What is the name for a muscle that assists the prime mover?

c) synergist

EXAMPLE QUESTIONS: ANSWERS FOR REVIEW cont.

3.10 What is the name for a muscle that performs the main action?

   a) agonist

3.11 Which movements are associated with the sagittal plane?

   d) flexion and extension

3.12 What is the name of the movement of the foot when the toes point down?

   c) plantar flexion

 NOTES

EXAMPLE QUESTIONS: ANSWERS FOR REVIEW

4 Cartilage, ligaments and tendons

4.1 What type of cartilage covers the end of a bone?

c) articular

4.2 What type of cartilage can be found in the nose and ear?

b) elastic

4.3 What type of cartilage can be found between vertebral bodies?

a) fibro

4.4 What color is articular cartilage?

b) bluey-white

4.5 What is the main function of articular cartilage?

c) prevent friction

4.6 What type of cartilage gets lubricated by synovial fluid?

c) articular

4.7 What is the main function of fibro cartilage?

a) shock absorption

4.8 What is the main function of elastic cartilage?

b) support

4.9 Which type of tissue connects bone to bone?

c) ligament

EXAMPLE QUESTIONS: ANSWERS FOR REVIEW cont.

4.10 Which type of tissue connects muscle to bone?

b) tendon

4.11 What is the name of the fibro cartilage in the knee joint?

d) meniscus

4.12 Which type of tissue does the statement 'allows wanted but prevents unwanted movement' relate to?

c) ligament

 NOTES

EXAMPLE QUESTIONS: ANSWERS FOR REVIEW

5 The nervous and endocrine systems

5.1 Chemical messengers called hormones are secreted into the bloodstream from groups of cells known as what?

c) glands

5.2 Where are neurotransmitters secreted from?

a) nerve endings

5.3 What do the the brain, the brainstem and the spinal cord make up?

b) central nervous system

5.4 What is the series of nerve branches that lead into and away from the CNS known as?

a) peripheral nervous system

5.5 Which of the following receptors sense position?

a) proprioceptors

5.6 Which of the following receptors sense pain?

c) nociceptors

5.7 Which of the following receptors sense temperature?

d) thermoreceptors

5.8 Which of the following receptors sense chemical composition?

b) chemoreceptors

EXAMPLE QUESTIONS: ANSWERS FOR REVIEW cont.

5.9 Cortisol and noradrenaline are secreted by which gland?

d) adrenals

5.10 Blood calcium levels are regulated by which gland?

b) parathyroid

5.11 Insulin is secreted by which gland?

c) pancreas

5.12 Cortisol, testosterone and estrogen belong to a group of hormones known as what?

d) steroid hormones

 NOTES

EXAMPLE QUESTIONS: ANSWERS FOR REVIEW

6 Energy systems

6.1 When a phosphate molecule is reattached to ADP to make ATP, what is the process called?

d) resynthesis

6.2 The 'powerhouse' within a muscle cell where ATP is generated aerobically is known as the what?

b) mitochondria

6.3 What is anaerobic glycolysis?

b) breaking down glucose without the presence of oxygen

6.4 What is aerobic glycolysis?

a) breaking down glucose in the presence of oxygen

6.5 Which of the following is given off as a by-product of aerobic glycolysis?

d) carbon dioxide and water

6.6 Which of the following is given off as a by-product of anaerobic glycolysis?

c) lactic acid

6.7 Which of the following is produced as a result of the incomplete breakdown of fat due to lack of available carbohydrate?

c) ketones

6.8 Which energy system contributes the most (in percentage terms) at the start of exercise?

c) ATP–CP

EXAMPLE QUESTIONS: ANSWERS FOR REVIEW cont.

6.9 Which energy system contributes the least (in percentage terms) at the start of exercise?

d) aerobic (fat)

6.10 Which energy system contributes the most (in percentage terms) in short-sprint events such as the 100 meters?

c) ATP–CP

6.11 Which energy system contributes the most (in percentage terms) in events such as the 800 meters?

b) aerobic glycolysis

6.12 Which energy system contributes the most (in percentage terms) in events such as jogging?

b) aerobic (fat)

 NOTES

EXAMPLE QUESTIONS: ANSWERS FOR REVIEW

7 The heart and the circulatory system

7.1 The heart muscle is also known as what?

d) myocardium

7.2 The heart muscle is covered on the inside by a layer of tissue known as what?

a) endocardium

7.3 The entire heart muscle is covered on the outside by a layer of fibrous tissue known as what?

c) pericardium

7.4 The mitral valve is otherwise known as the what?

c) bicuspid

7.5 The sinoatrial node can be found in which chamber of the heart?

a) right atrium

7.6 The aortic valve can be found in which chamber of the heart?

d) left ventricle

7.7 The amount of blood pumped out of the ventricles each beat is known as what?

c) stroke volume

7.8 The amount of blood pumped out of the ventricles each beat, multiplied by the heart rate in beats per minute, is known as what?

b) cardiac output

EXAMPLE QUESTIONS: ANSWERS FOR REVIEW cont.

7.9 The amount of blood left in the ventricles after each beat is known as what?

  a) end diastolic volume

7.10 Erythrocyte is another name for what?

  a) red blood cell

7.11 Leukocyte is another name for what?

  b) white blood cell

7.12 Which of the following makes up the largest percentage of volume in the blood?

  c) plasma

 NOTES

EXAMPLE QUESTIONS: ANSWERS FOR REVIEW

8 The respiratory system

8.1 Air sacs in the lungs are also known as what?

  a) alveoli

8.2 The double membrane surrounding the lungs is known as what?

  b) pleura

8.3 Gaseous exchange takes place between what?

  a) alveoli and capillaries

8.4 What is the percentage difference of oxygen between inspired and expired air?

  c) 5

8.5 The amount of air left in the lungs after a maximal expiration is known as what?

  c) residual volume

8.6 The maximum amount of air breathed out of the lungs after a maximum breath in is known as what?

  d) vital capacity

8.7 Which of the following gases can stimulate breathing when blood levels reach a certain point?

  b) carbon dioxide

8.8 The amount of air taken into the lungs during a normal breath is called what?

  b) tidal volume

EXAMPLE QUESTIONS: ANSWERS FOR REVIEW cont.

8.9 The voice box is otherwise known as what?

a) larynx

8.10 The windpipe is otherwise known as what?

c) trachea

8.11 Which of the following lead directly into the alveoli?

d) bronchiole

8.12 Which of the following structures is only one cell thick?

d) capillaries

 NOTES

EXAMPLE QUESTIONS: ANSWERS FOR REVIEW

9 Core stability

9.1 Muscles that provide constant periods of tension in a postural role are otherwise known as what type of muscle?

d) tonic

9.2 Muscles that provide brief periods of tension in a strength role are otherwise known as what type of muscle?

c) phasic

9.3 Which of the following can be considered to be predominantly stabilizing muscles for the core?

b) multifidus, transversus abdominis, diaphragm

9.4 Which of the following can be considered to be predominantly mobilizing muscles for the core?

c) erector spinae, rectus abdominis, external obliques

9.5 Which of the following can be considered to be predominantly a stabilizing muscle for the hip joint?

d) gluteus medius

9.6 Which of the following can be considered to be predominantly a mobilizing muscle for the hip joint?

b) gluteus maximus

9.7 When local muscles contract to compress the 'fluid ball' in the abdomen it is known as what?

b) intra-abdominal pressure

EXAMPLE QUESTIONS: ANSWERS FOR REVIEW cont.

9.8 An increase in the tension of the connective tissues in the spinal region is known as what?

d) thoracolumbar fascia gain

9.9 Research has suggested that what minimum percentage of maximum contraction is sufficient to create sufficient intra-abdominal pressure to stabilize the spine?

d) 30

9.10 What best relates to the following statement – *'when there is minimal force placed on the spine and the structures that surround it such as tendons, cartilage and ligaments.'*?

b) neutral zone

9.11 True or false? Normal screening procedures should be carried out prior to prescribing core stabilization exercises, but those with back problems should be excluded.

True

9.12 The length of time, number of repetitions and frequency of practice of conscious contraction required to develop subconscious contraction control of the transversus abdominis can take up to how long?

d) a few months

NOTES

EXAMPLE QUESTIONS: ANSWERS FOR REVIEW

10 Components and principles of fitness

10.1 The ACSM defines what as '*an ability to perform daily activities with vigor and the demonstration of traits and capacities that are associated with a low risk of premature development of hypokinetic diseases*'?

c) health-related physical fitness

10.2 The World Health Organization defines what as '*a state of complete physical, mental and social well-being and not merely the absence of disease or infirmity*'?

a) wellness

10.3 The ACSM defines what as '*a set of attributes that people have or achieve that relates to the ability to perform physical activity*'?

b) physical fitness

10.4 VO_{2max} is measured in what?

c) $mLO_2.kg^{-1}min^{-1}$

10.5 An increase in intensity that results in an equal increase in heart rate has what kind of relationship?

a) linear

10.6 What is the term used to define an increase in muscle cross section?

c) hypertrophy

10.7 What is the term used to define a decrease in muscle cross section?

b) atrophy

EXAMPLE QUESTIONS: ANSWERS FOR REVIEW cont.

10.8 What is the term used to describe the perception of soreness in a muscle in the period shortly following intense exercise training?

a) DOMS

10.9 The type of stretching that involves the use of a partner is known as what?

d) PNF

10.10 The type of stretching that predominantly involves the use of momentum and gravity is known as what?

b) ballistic

10.11 Which of the following formulae can be used to calculate BMI?

b) weight/height^2

10.12 In relation to BMI, what figure is classed as obese?

b) over 30

 NOTES

EXAMPLE QUESTIONS: ANSWERS FOR REVIEW

11 Screening for exercise and safety issues

11.1 The PAR-Q is a screening questionnaire used to identify conditions prior to encouraging exercise at what level?

    c) a light-to-moderate intensity

11.2 How long is the PAR-Q valid for?

    d) 12 months

11.3 True or false? The PAR-Q is a confidential document.

    True

11.4 Which of the following is classed as a risk factor in relation to family history?

    b) myocardial infarction or sudden death before age 55 in father, brother or son; before age 65 in mother, sister or daughter

11.5 Which of the following is classed as a risk factor in relation to hypertension?

    d) systolic pressure of 140 mmHg or above, or diastolic pressure of 90 mmHg or above

11.6 Which of the following is classed as a risk factor in relation to obesity?

    d) BMI of 30 kg/m^2 or above

11.7 Which of the following is classed as a risk factor in relation to dyslipidemia?

    c) total serum cholesterol of more than 5.2 mmol/l

11.8 Which of the following is classed as a risk factor in relation to dyslipidemia?

    a) LDL more than 3.4 mmol/l, or HDL less than 1.03 mmol/l

EXAMPLE QUESTIONS: ANSWERS FOR REVIEW cont.

11.9 With regard to risk stratification, the ACSM states that which group of people is at moderate risk?

c) men 45 or older and women 55 or older or those with two or more risk factors

11.10 Which of the following is classed as a risk factor in relation to impaired fasting glucose?

c) 100 mg/dl or more

11.11 With regard to risk stratification, which group of people does the ACSM classify as low risk?

c) men under 45 years and women under 55 years who are asymptomatic and have no more than one risk factor

11.12 True or false? A sedentary lifestyle is classed as a risk factor for coronary heart disease.

True

 NOTES

EXAMPLE QUESTIONS: ANSWERS FOR REVIEW

12 Behavioral change and goal setting

12.1 The 'Stages of Change' model follows what type of pattern?
   b) cyclical

12.2 Approximately what percentage of all individuals will experience relapse back to the contemplation or precontemplation stage?
   c) 15 percent

12.3 True or false? Cognitive processes are usually adopted by individuals in the early stages of the 'Stages of Change' model, from not thinking about exercise to taking up exercise.
   True

12.4 True or false? Behavioral processes are usually adopted by individuals in the later stages of the 'Stages of Change' model.
   True

12.5 What is the following a definition of: 'the internal mechanisms and external stimuli that arouse and direct our behavior.'?
   d) motivation

12.6 Which term is used to describe an individual being motivated to exercise by factors such as enjoyment, fun or self-satisfaction?
   a) intrinsic motivation

12.7 When a skill is broken down into manageable units that the subject can focus on, it is known as what type of goal?
   c) process

EXAMPLE QUESTIONS: ANSWERS FOR REVIEW cont.

12.8 Goals that are concerned only with the ultimate outcome, for example success or failure, winning or losing, are known as what type of goal?

    b) outcome

12.9 In the acronym SMARTER, what does the first R stand for?

    c) realistic

12.10 In the acronym SMARTER, what does the M stand for?

    b) measurable

12.11 In the acronym SMARTER, what does the S stand for?

    b) specific

12.12 In the acronym SMARTER, what does the A stand for?

    a) adjustable

NOTES

EXAMPLE QUESTIONS: ANSWERS FOR REVIEW

13 Components and induction of an exercise session

13.1 According to the ACSM, what period of time is recommended for a warm-up?

b) 5–10 minutes

13.2 According to the ACSM, what intensity of exercise, related to heart rate maximum, is recommended for the cardiovascular endurance component?

c) 55–90 percent

13.3 In relation to cardio training zones, what range of heart rate maximum is the weight-management zone?

b) 60–70 percent

13.4 In relation to cardio training zones, what range of heart rate maximum is the aerobic zone?

c) 70–80 percent

13.5 In relation to cardio training zones, what range of heart rate maximum is the anaerobic zone?

d) 80–90 percent

13.6 What type of training is otherwise known as 'speed play'?

d) fartlek

13.7 Which cycle of periodization is usually associated with a seven-day period?

b) microcycle

13.8 Which cycle of periodization is usually associated with a period of a few weeks?

c) mesocycle

EXAMPLE QUESTIONS: ANSWERS FOR REVIEW cont.

13.9 Which cycle of periodization is usually associated with a 12-month period?

d) macrocycle

13.10 What is the acronym NAMSIT used for?

b) induction for resistance machines

13.11 What is the acronym IDEA used for?

a) induction for cardiovascular machines

13.12 Which of the following cardiovascular machines is normally associated with higher impact?

c) treadmill

 NOTES

EXAMPLE QUESTIONS: ANSWERS FOR REVIEW

14 Monitoring exercise intensity

14.1 What is the formula for predicted maximum heart rate?

   c) 220 – age

14.2 True or false? Predicted maximum heart rate has an error of up to plus or minus 12 beats per minute.

   True

14.3 True or false? A graded maximum heart rate test should be used on all individuals to find their maximum heart rate.

   False

14.4 What is the predicted maximum heart rate for a 39-year-old person?

   b) 181 bpm

14.5 What is 70 percent of the predicted maximum heart rate for a 20-year-old person?

   c) 140 bpm

14.6 What is 80 percent of the predicted maximum heart rate for a 40-year-old person?

   a) 144 bpm

14.7 What is 55 percent of the predicted maximum heart rate for a 40-year-old person?

   d) 99 bpm

14.8 What is the equivalent value of 1 MET?

   c) $3.5 \ mlO_2.kg^{-1}min^{-1}$

EXAMPLE QUESTIONS: ANSWERS FOR REVIEW cont.

14.9 What is the equivalent value of 1 MET?

a) 1.0 kcal.kg⁻¹hr⁻¹

14.10 How many kilocalories would an 80 kg person expend in 30 minutes doing an exercise valued at 10 METs?

b) 400

14.11 How many kilocalories would a 60 kg person expend in two hours and 30 minutes doing an exercise valued at 8 METs?

c) 1,200

14.12 Which of the following statements is most accurate in regard to the definition of 12RM?

d) A weight that can be lifted 12 times and not 13 times

 NOTES

INDEX
